SPORTS NUTRITION GUIDE

Minerals, Vitamins & Antioxidants for Athletes

Dr. Michael COLGAN

www.applepublishing.com

The Information contained in this book was prepared from medical and scientific sources which are referenced herein and are believed to be accurate and reliable. However, the opinions expressed herein by the author do not necessarily represent the opinions or the views of the publisher. Nor should the information herein be used to treat or to prevent any medical condition unless it is used with the full knowledge, compliance and agreement of our personal physician or other licensed health care professional. Readers are strongly advised to seek the advice of their personal health care professional(s) before proceeding with any changes in any health care program.

National Library of Canada Cataloguing in Publication Data

Colgan, Michael
        Sports nutrition guide

ISBN 0-9695272-8-4

        **1. Athletes—Nutrition. 2. Vitamins in human nutrition.
        3. Minerals in human nutrition. I. Title.**

TX361.A8C582 2002   613.2'8   C2002-900956-1

Apple Publishing Company Ltd.
220 East 59th Avenue
Vancouver, British Columbia
Canada V5X 1X9 Tel: (604) 214-6688   Fax: (604) 214-3566

E-mail: books@applepublishing.com   Website: www.applepublishing.com

10   9   8   7   6   5   4   3   2

INTRODUCTION

Eight exciting years have passed since I wrote *Optimum Sports Nutrition*[1] which, became somewhat of a nutrition standard for athletes. This new book continues our quest for excellence with the amazing new discoveries in sports nutrition. I can share with you only a fraction of the 8,000 plus research papers published from 1995 to today. But I'll do my damnedest to cover enough of them to enable you to design a personal nutrition program that will give your body all the materials it needs to excel.

The latest discoveries in sports nutrition show clearly that the old Recommended Dietary Allowances (RDA), formulated primarily to prevent deficiency diseases in sedentary folk,[1-3] have no relevance for athletes.[4-6] Nor do the recent Daily Recommended Intakes (DRI), or Daily Values (DV), which are essentially the old RDA, in a garish new waistcoat.[7,8] And the even newer, Recommended Daily Intakes (RDI), and Estimated Average Requirements (EAR), are simply further pedantic extensions of the same old *minimal* nutrition. You can safely ignore them. They do not incorporate most of the new science, and do not even address the nutritional quest of athletes, and focus of this book – to discover the parameters of *optimal* nutrition?

The new nutrition science also soundly condemns the processed pap, masquerading as food, that fills fast-food franchises and crowds supermarket shelves. Confused by slick advertising, however, in which the best of American bodies are handsomely paid to pretend they grew from eating garbage, the majority of Americans, continue to gobble processed pap as their major food source.[9-11]

And numerous confused "health professionals", continue to recommend the pap as the only nutrition you need. As you will see from the evidence ahead, those who do so are probably similarly confused about the relative whereabouts of the arse and the elbow.

If you want to excel in sport, you will reject both pap and RDI, and instead put your trust in science. I am confident in the new science, not only because of the meticulous research, but also because we have used it at the Colgan Institute to help hundreds of athletes develop into champions, over the whole alphabet of sport from archery to yachting. It will work equally well for you, whether you are bound for Olympic glory, a worthy weekend warrior, or simply a stubborn old coot like me still pushing to heights long dreamed. Seize this science today and go for all the gusto!

- Michael Colgan

OTHER BOOKS by Dr. COLGAN

- *NEW NUTRITION*
- *HORMONAL HEALTH*
- *BEAT ARTHRITIS*
- *PROTECT YOUR PROSTATE*
- *NEW POWER PROGRAM*
- *YOU CAN PREVENT CANCER*
- *PROGRESS HEALTH SERIES (6 booklets)*
- *COLGANChronicles (Newsletter)*

For more information, visit www.applepublishing.com

The above titles are available at special quantity discounts for bulk purchase for sales promotions, premiums, fund-raising, and education needs. Special books or book excerpts also can be created to fit specific needs. For details, telephone (604) 214-6688 or fax (604) 214-3566 or email books@applepublishing.com

Table of CONTENTS

1

ONE SYSTEM OF CHEMISTRY

Athletes tend to be independent, self-reliant individuals. But these desirable traits also predispose them to think they are separate from the world, in complete control of their bodies, each cozy and secure in a little skin bag. If you believe that, I have a guaranteed method to leap tall buildings that might interest you too.

To gain the athletic edge, you need to realize that you are no more than a localized bit of the mass of solids, liquids, gases, and vibrations that flow around you and through you every living day. The world, including you, is all one single system of chemistry. Changes in that chemistry, whether they occur inside your skin or outside in the environment, completely determine what you think, what you feel, and how well you are able to perform. Even your most secret beliefs, are little more than a reflection of the ongoing chemistry inside you and out in your surroundings.

You are constructed from a mix of natural chemicals that have formed part of the Earth since life began. Science can track the beneficial chemicals that construct your body, and the detrimental chemicals that damage it, through the soil, through the air, through the plants and animals we use for food, through you, and back to the soil again.

The science of sports nutrition consists of designing your individual nutrition, training, and lifestyle, so that your body can retain and use sufficient of the beneficial chemicals, and avoid or expel the detrimental. The first step is to realize that *you and your environment are one single interacting system of chemistry.*

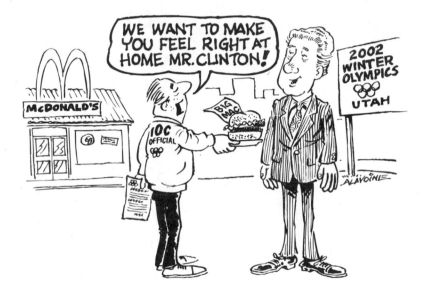

You Are Recycled

You should also know where you are coming from. In the Archaen era, 400 million years ago, a miraculous combination of gases produced a few simple bacteria. Physicists, including my late mentor, Nobel Laureate Dick Feynman of MIT, consider that it could not have been a random event. A hand of intelligence reached into the chaos, and the evolution of life began.

At that time the atmosphere was mainly carbon dioxide with a little methane and nitrogen, but almost no oxygen. Over countless millennia the Archaen bacteria multiplied across the face of the Earth. They absorbed the carbon dioxide and excreted oxygen as a waste product. Gradually the atmosphere changed so that plants could survive. Vast forests grew up and consumed the carbon dioxide and excreted oxygen at a prodigious rate. Carbon dioxide declined to its present 0.09% of the atmosphere, and oxygen increased to its present 21%, making possible the evolution of human life.

The next step in understanding the body and its needs is to ask: what is human life made of? As Table 1 shows, the body is 99.9% gaseous and mineral elements. Your 65 % of oxygen comes from the air as a waste product of plants. Most of the rest of your oxygen, plus your 10% of hydrogen, comes from the water you drink. And the carbon, calcium and other minerals come from the plants you eat, either directly or through the animals we use as food. All the other minerals, all the vitamins, and all other nutrients make up less than 0.1% of your flesh.

Table 1 shows clearly that the usual emphasis on vitamins as primary nutrients is entirely wrong. The primary nutrients are the gaseous and mineral elements. That is why this book places minerals first in the title. You and I are almost entirely recycled products made from a mix of ancient elements that have been used over and over again for countless millennia. Unless we get these main chunks of our flesh right first, taking mineral and vitamin pills is a waste of time, because there is no way they can correct, or compensate for, basic faults in the bulk of the mix.

Table 1:
Composition of the Human Body

Gaseous Elements	% of Human Body
Oxygen	65 %
Hydrogen	10 %
Nitrogen	3 %
Total	**78 %**
Major Mineral Elements	
Carbon	18.5 %
Calcium	1.2 %
Phosphorus	1.0 %
Minor Mineral Elements	
Potassium, Sulfur, Sodium Chloride, Magnesium	1.2 %
Total	**99.9 %**
Trace elements, vitamins and all other nutrients	0.1%
Total	**100%**

Every molecule of your flesh has lived on Earth before. Every element has been through the guts of millions of creatures before you. The calcium of your bones was digested by ancient sea creatures and grown into their shells, which then degraded into the soils from which the plants and animals we use as food obtain their calcium.

Most of the sulfur in the proteins that comprise half the dry weight of your body, is the dimethyl sulfide excrement of a minute phytoplankton called ***Emiliana huxleyii***, which blooms in uncountable profusion over thousands of square miles of oceans every day. The excrement rises in evaporation of the ocean surface to seed the clouds with sulfur, which then float over the land and return the sulfur to the soil in rain. Without *Emiliana*, most of humankind would sicken and die.[1]

Step by tiny step, over four million years the human body evolved, by learning to convert a precise mixture of these recycled natural chemicals of the Earth, into muscles, bones, glands, organs and brain. These chemicals we now call "nutrients." The interactions of these nutrients determine your structure, your intelligence, your emotions, your athletic ability, all the stuff that you call "I."

For its construction during evolution, the human body could use only the chemicals that were available at the time. For each of these chemicals it grew incredibly precise mechanisms to use it in myriad ways. These ancient chemicals of the Earth are the only substances your body has had sufficient evolutionary time to learn to use correctly. They are the *only* chemicals that it can use today to produce optimum function.

For optimum function, therefore, you should *put inside your body only those ancient nutrients, which have been present on Earth for millions of years, those unique substances upon which the bodies of our ancestors evolved.*

First Principle of Sports Nutrition
Design your diet so that you take into your body only those ancient nutrients upon which humankind evolved.

*"See first that the design is
wise and just;
that ascertained, pursue it
resolutely;
do not for one repulse forego
the purpose that you resolved
to effect."*

- William Shakespeare

Minerals Elements *(cont)*

Chromium (picolinate)	200 - 800 mcg
Selenium (l-selenomethionine)	100 - 600 mcg
Manganese (aspartate, gluconate)	5 - 30 mg
Molybdenium (ammonium molybdate)	100 - 300 mcg
Silicon (popularly called silica)	10 - 30 mg
Boron (citrate, aspartate)	3 - 10 mg
Colbalt	As part of B$_{12}$ complex
Vanadium (vanadyl sulfate)	25 - 100 mcg
Fluroide	Food and fluoridated water
Arsenic	Food sources only
Nickel**	Food sources only
Tin**	Food sources only

Vitamins

Vitamin A (palmitate)	3,000 - 10,000 IU
Beta-Carotene	10,000 - 50,000 IU
Vitamin B$_1$, thiamin	10 - 150 mg
Vitamin B$_2$, riboflavin	10 - 100 mg
Vitamin B$_3$, niacin	25 - 50 mg
Vitamin B$_3$, niacinamide	20 - 100 mg
Vitamin B$_6$, pyridoxine	15 - 75 mg
Vitamin B$_{12}$, cyanocobalamin	25 - 250 mcg
Folate (folic acid)	400 - 2000 mcg
Biotin	600 - 5000 mcg
Pantothenic acid	20 - 650 mg
Vitamin C, ascorbic acid	500 - 4000 mg
Vitamin C, calcium ascorbate	250 - 1000 mg
Vitamin C, magnesium ascorbate	100 - 500 mg
Vitamin C, ascorbyl palmitate	50 - 250 mg
Vitamin D, cholecalciferol	400 - 800 IU
Vitamin E, d-alpha tocopherol, mixed tocopherols	700 - 2600 IU
Vitamin K, phylloquinone	100 - 200 mcg

Adjunctive Nutrients

Co-enzyme Q10	30 - 100 mg
L-glutathione	50 - 200 mg
N-acetyl-cysteine	100 - 400 mg

**Probably essential mineral

Adjunctive Nutrients *(cont)*

L-glutamine	1000 - 4000 mg
L-methionine	500 - 1000 mg
Acetyl-l-carnitine	100 - 400 mg
Taurine	100 - 300 mg
Arginine alpha-ketoglutarate	1000 - 10,000 mg
L-tyrosine	500 - 2000 mg
Choline	100 - 300 mg
Phosphatidylcholine	200 - 1000 mg
Phosphatidylserine	100 - 800 mg
Alpha-lipoic acid	100 - 400 mg
Sodium bicarbonate	1000 - 5000 mg
Inositol	100 - 300 mg
Para-amino-benzoic acid	10 - 50 mg
Pyrroloquinoline quinone	5 - 20 mg
Melatonin	1.0 - 4.0 mg
S-adenosylmethionine	200 - 600 mg
Creatine monohydrate	1000 - 5000 mg
Glucosamine sulfate	500 - 3000 mg
Chondroitin sulfate	200 - 500 mg
Flavanones	100 - 500 mg
Methyl-allyl-trisulfide	300 - 1000 mg
Lycopene	20 - 100 mg
Lutein	10 - 50 mg
Procyanadins	100 - 200 mg
Catechins	10 - 40 mg
Bioflavones	10 - 20 mg
Indoles	10 - 100 mg
Anthocyanosides	10 - 50 mg
Anthocyanins	10 - 25 mg
Flavonolignans	10 - 100 mg
Isoflavones	10 - 100 mg
Coumarins	10 - 50 mg
Saw palmetto	200 - 600 mg
Urtica	500 - 1000 mg
Pygeum	300 - 800 mg

+Colgan Institute, San Diego, 2001
**Probably essential mineral

2

SYNERGY

Nutrients never work alone. The chemistry of your body is so precise that if even one essential nutrient is deficient, the whole mixture becomes defective and optimal function is impossible. You need only microscopic amounts of some substances, but every one of them is essential to the integrity of the mix.

Your body works well on only a few micrograms (millionths of a gram) of vitamin B_{12}, for example. But if you become deficient in B_{12}, your energy declines immediately, you cannot make healthy red blood cells, and you develop the disease of pernicious anemia. Without sufficient B_{12} in the mix, none of the other nutrients can work properly. Left untreated, B_{12} deficiency gradually destroys your brain, leading to insanity and certain death, all for the want of a daily amount of a vitamin so minute you could hardly see it on the head of a pin.[1]

In the sports marketplace, where a myriad of incomplete mineral and vitamin supplements each claims to be the best and only, you must guard your body well with the principle of synergy. *It is the interaction of all essential nutrients together, which determines optimum biological function*.

Essential Nutrients

To help you get all the nutrients you need, Table 2 sets out the ranges of daily requirements for athletes that the Colgan Institute has derived from the research literature and our own studies over the last 26 years. Because of new discoveries, it contains numerous substances that were not listed in my 1993 book.[2] The table reflects the state of nutrition science today.

Table 2:
Daily Ranges of Nutrients Require to Provide Complete Nutrition for Athletes[+]

Water *See Volume 2*	2 - 4 litres/day
Proteins *See Volume 2*	60 - 240 grams
Carbohydrates *See Volume 2*	100 - 400 grams
Essential Fats *See Volume 2*	40 - 160 grams
Minerals Elements	
Oxygen (gas, liquid and solid)	Supplied by air and water
Hydrogen (gas. liquid and solid)	Supplied by air, water & carbohydrates
Nitrogen (gas and solid)	Supplied mainly by protein foods
Carbon	Base structure of all food
Calcium (carbonate, citrate, ascorbate)	1000 - 2000 mg
Phosphorus (potassium, phosphate)	300 - 1000 mg
Potassium (phosphate, bicarbonate)	500 - 1000 mg
Sulfur (methyl-sulfonyl-methane)	1000 - 6000 mg
Sodium	Food sources supply excess
Chloride	Food sources supply excess
Magnesium (aspartate, ascorbate)	400 - 1800 mg
Iron (picolinate)	15 - 40 mg
Zinc (picolinate)	15 - 50 mg
Copper (gluconate)	1 - 3 mg
Iodine (potassium iodide)	150 - 300 mcg

[+]Colgan Institute, San Diego, 2001

The ranges of nutrient amounts in Table 2 are those which we have found to yield the best long-term results with athletes. They bear little relation to the old RDA[3], or the new RDI,[1,4] derived from the RDA, which are point estimates of the amounts of nutrients required to prevent certain deficiency diseases in sedentary people. Although the RDI are quoted extensively in the food and nutrition literature as an ideal, Dr A E Harper, former Chairman of the RDA Committee, stressed on numerous occasions that RDA, "are not recommendations for the ideal diet" and "do not represent optimal requirements".[5]

Because of the degradation of our soils and our food,[6] Table 2 also bears little relation to the meager nutrient supply that you can obtain from even an excellent diet. In 1998, after 57 years of denial, the Food and Nutrition Board of the US National Academy of Sciences, finally admitted that the American food supply is deficient in nutrients, and recommended that most Americans take vitamin/mineral supplements.[7]

I'm pleased to see that the National Academy of Sciences message is getting across. A representative recent study of American athletes in 22 universities found that more than 50% take supplements.[8] So do two-thirds of the tough, fit guys applying for entry to the US Special Forces and Ranger training schools, compared with less than one-third of Joe Averages.[9] Supplement users in general are also leaner, more active, better educated, and non-smokers.[10] Smart folk.

So many incomplete and poorly bioavailable supplements flood the marketplace, however, that many athletes taking them are still deficient.[2,11-14] Table 2 guides you past these problems, by giving not only the complete list of essential nutrients, but also the range of amounts that covers genetic and other individual differences in athletes. The table also gives the best commercially available chemical form of each nutrient.

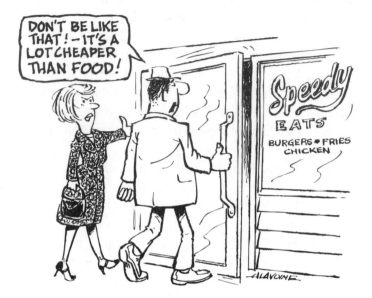

Adjunctive Nutrients

Table 2 also contains a list labeled Adjunctive Nutrients. We call them "adjunctive" because they are not included in official government lists of essential nutrients. Are they then unnecessary? To answer that question you need to know a little history about the shifting nature of "essential".

In the early 20th century, the term "essential nutrients" was decreed to mean certain chemicals that the human body cannot make, but has to obtain from food, and which also act as coenzymes for essential enzyme functions. These nutrients were discovered by depriving experimental subjects of each one separately, and watching for the development of deficiency diseases.

Seemed logical at the time, but Nature has a habit of upsetting human decrees. Let's take a few examples. After a decade or so, along came discoveries of **vitamins A, C, D, and E**, which must be obtained from food, but do not act in the body primarily as coenzymes. Authorities had to shift the goalposts.

A second example is the essential mineral chromium. In 1968, the US RDA Committee of the American Academy of Sciences solemnly dismissed **chromium** as unnecessary for human nutrition.[15] But, by 1980 the evidence was overwhelming that chromium is essential for insulin metabolism. The goalposts shifted once more.[16]

Delayed by similar bureaucratic fuddling, it took 35 years of evidence before the mineral **selenium** was admitted into the sacred US RDA list in 1989.[3] Some governments, such as of New Zealand, however, are so far behind the science, they still restrict access to selenium supplements today, in 2001. Yet New Zealand soils and food are so deficient in selenium, that the average daily intake is only 28 micrograms per day,[17] less than half the US RDI of 70 micrograms. And selenium deficiency diseases are rampant.

Pantothenic acid, shown to be essential by the great nutrition scientist Roger Williams in 1939,[18] didn't make the US essential nutrients list until the advent of the RDI in 1995. **Coenzyme Q10, alpha-lipoic acid, choline, inositol**, and numerous other nutrients hover in limbo, because the body can make a little of them but probably not sufficient for good health.

The minerals **nickel, silicon** (popularly called silica), **boron**, and **vanadium** are almost certainly essential. So is a minute amount of **arsenic**, yes, arsenic, which we get in our food every day. And a host of polyphenols are showing their paces in coenzyme and other reactions, without which we would get very sick indeed. Table 2, which includes all of these nutrients, is based on the latest science not on political obfuscation.

Amounts Of Nutrients Required

The ranges and amounts of nutrients in Table 2 are much larger than recommendations of some dietitians and physicians, most of whom have never measured actual nutrient use in athletes. Some of these folk will object strongly to our ranges, by quoting research suggesting that the RDI are sufficient. So I want to make our criteria crystal clear.

First, science is still far, far away from determining optimal standards for nutrients. All that governments have to date is minimal standards, defined by the appearance of deficiency symptoms during short-term studies of a few weeks to a few months.[3] In trying to decide optima, **all** such studies are useless, because they are too short to allow for the minimum six months to one year turnover of body cells that would show superior function. Since adopting this cell

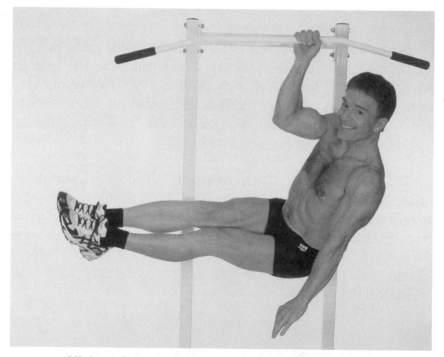

Michael Colgan at age 62, still following the path.

turnover criterion, the Colgan Institute has recorded dramatic improvements in function with long-term supplementation, because we have been able to study many hundreds of athletes who have been on our programs continuously for up to *20 years.*

Tests of Nutrition Status

The second problem with many nutrition experiments is the tests used to measure sufficiency. To listen to pronouncements of poorly informed health professionals, you would think that science has the testing of a person's nutrition status all sewn up. Not a chance! I pointed out the shortcomings of many of the tests in 1993.[2] And a recent scholarly collection of research on sports nutrition, edited by Professor Ira Wolinsky of the University of Houston and Professor Judy Driscoll of the University of Nebraska agreed that we are still a very long way from measuring optimal status.[19]

In a nutshell, there are few reliable tests of adequate nutritional status, and none at all of optimal nutritional status, except for extremely complex repeated biopsy procedures that are both invasive and time and cost prohibitive. All the one-hit, walk-in doctor's office vitamin and mineral tests now being touted across America, are about as accurate as dangling crystals over your head while chanting in Swahili.

Why am I so sure? Because I've spent 26 years trying every test in the book. Most tests are done using *extracellular* body fluids such as blood and urine. But nutrients function primarily *intracellularly*, and their concentrations in cells and organs can be hundreds of times higher than in the blood. Body fluids are mainly transport systems for nutrients, conveying them to their cellular sites of use. Measuring the amount of a nutrient in a blood test is like counting food trucks on the freeway for an hour to try to determine the amount of food in the city.

Even when you *can* measure nutrients intracellularly, such as red cell folate levels, you have the huge problem of which cells to use. Liver cells, brain cells, heart cells, blood cells all differ widely in their levels of different nutrients. And, even if you could find athletes silly enough to let you take cell samples from their hearts and brains, there is a huge range of variation in cellular levels of nutrients between apparently healthy individuals. What is the minimum healthy level for each type of cell? What is the optimal level? Science has hardly a clue.

The only way to test whether or not nutrient supplements improve health and performance, is long-term measurement of health and performance with and without supplementation. I conducted some of the first of these long studies in the early '80s, showing six-month improvements in strength and in marathon running.[20] Long studies didn't catch on at the time, because any research of more than a few weeks is very expensive, and the duration of most studies is decided by the size of the research grant. Since then, however, extended studies have become the gold standard, especially in medical research, because scientists have realized it is the only way to find out what the hell is happening.

This enlightened approach has produced a mass of new evidence showing that people under constant stress, especially athletes, need much larger amounts of nutrients than previously thought. We cover a lot of this recent work ahead. Suffice to say here, that any health professional who advises a good mixed diet, or at best a one-a-day vitamin, as adequate for athletes, is guilty of malpractice. Athletes advised to train on nutritional programs that fail to supply sufficient structural nutrients to offset training stresses, are put at constant risk of illness and injury.[21-28]

Worse, there is considerable new evidence that the intensity of training and competition today, often practiced under insufficient nutrition, may predispose athletes to premature degenerative disease in later life, including neck, back, hip, knee, and ankle disease and dementia.[29-34] Our own records show tantalizing suggestions but insufficient cases yet to prove them, that overtraining combined with inadequate nutrition, may predispose the athlete to subsequent development of heart disease, cancer and premature degeneration of the brain.

As this book goes to press, the media are reporting a new form of heart disease, Stone's Syndrome. It is named after actress Sharon Stone, who suffered a stroke in a healthy heart purely from the effects of intensive exercise and inadequate food intake. More telling examples may be champion miler Steve Scott who developed testicular cancer, and New Zealand's John Walker who developed Parkinson's.

Second Principle of Sports Nutrition
Nutrients Work Only in Synergy.
Design your diet so that you receive a complete and proportionate mix of all the nutrients every day.

"If you have no time for complete and balanced nutrition, you better reserve a lot of time for illness."
- *Michael Colgan*
Lecture Series, 2000

3

NATURE MADE ALL THE LOCKS

I want to stress again how closely all of us are bound to Nature. Optimum function of your body is totally dependent on ingestion of the right mix of naturally occurring chemicals in your air, your water and your food. Screw around with them, and they will screw around with you.

The arrogance of 20th century technology obscured this basic principle of life on Earth. Unthinking scientists claimed to design better chemicals than those of Nature. And ignorant health and environmental bureaucrats, hell-bent on "progress" and profits, foisted these chemicals upon an unwitting public, in the air, in the water, in the food and ploughed into the fields. In the 1960's, Rachel Carson's **Silent Spring** informed the public only too well of the greed and mendacity of agribusiness.[1] So virulent were the poisons poured upon the crops, they killed every living thing for miles around, including thousands of farm workers. Today the exact same action would rightly be called bioterrorism, and spark a National Emergency that would make Usama Bin Laden's treachery seem like a damp squib. Even now in "enlightened" 2002, mother's milk in the breast is badly polluted with DDT, PCBs and the much more toxic polychlorodiben-zo-dioxins (PCDDs) which pass to and poison the baby. This breast milk pollution has worsened during the 1990s, to such an extent, it would be a felony to transport the milk across a state line in any other container.[2,3]

Even the ancient nutrients that make up your flesh have not escaped the meddling of man's simian fingers. Vitamin E provides a telling example. Natural-source vitamin E, **d-alpha-tocopherol**, is usually extracted from soybeans. The "d" stands for "dextrorotatory" a right-hand twist of the molecule. This twist is the precise chemical key that fits your body locks for vitamin E in your nutrient transport system and in your cell membranes. So your body can use it well.

In contrast, man-made vitamin E, **dl-alpha-tocopherol**, is a mix of two synthetic chemicals, trimethylhydroquinone and isophytol. Only about 12% of it is "d," the right chemical key for your body. Nearly 90% of it is "l" for "levorotatory" a left-hand twist of the molecule. It does not fit your body locks. Consequently, the synthetic vitamin E still sold in the majority of pharmacies and health food stores has low biological activity, is poorly transported and quickly excreted from the body. It is next to useless for human nutrition.[4]

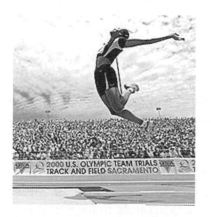

Marion Jones in the long jump showing that humans really can fly.

I feel optimistic nevertheless, about the future because, as only seems fitting, many of the health bureaucrats responsible for today's environmental mess are dead or dying prematurely by their own hand. The better educated and therefore humbler scientists that are rising to prominence today, are gradually coming to realize that *Nature made all the locks, and holds all the keys.*

Prescription Drugs Are Toxic

The best example of the toxicity of man-made molecules is prescription drugs. These chemicals are all man-made and never existed on Earth before the 20th century. Why have they grown to such prominence? One reason is the futile arrogance that man can design better than Nature. A second is our archaic laws, which decree that you cannot patent naturally occurring chemicals. Without patent protection there is little profit in selling them as prescription medicines. To make their chop, pharmaceutical companies have to throw man-made wrinkles into the chemistry, wrinkles that wreak havoc with nature's design of man.

All this stupidity occurred in the last 100 years. But evolution takes millennia. So the human body has had no time at all in evolutionary terms, to develop the mechanisms to deal with man-made drugs. They were not on Earth during human evolution, and are mostly invisible to the body's defensive chemistry. Although they have potent effects in reducing surface symptoms of disease, every man-made drug is toxic to the human system.

I have space for just one example. In 1998 the Journal of the American Medical Association published the figures for toxic effects of prescription drugs for one year for hospitals alone. Hospitals were chosen because they have precise records and control of drug prescription and use. These toxic effects were not errors in drug type or dosage. They were side-effects of drugs prescribed and given in accord with "good practice", as detailed in the *Physicians Desk Reference.* 2,216,000 patients in American hospitals were injured by drugs and 106,000 *died* of those injuries. This death toll dwarfs the 45,000 people per year killed in motor vehicle accidents. **Drugs prescribed in American hospitals are now our fourth leading cause of death.**[5]

In your quest for athletic success, make a clear distinction between the chemicals that form part of Nature's magnificent design, and the synthetic chemicals concocted by the puny hand of man.

Before you put anything into your body, always ask yourself this question. *Was this substance present during evolution, so that the human structure had time to develop the precise locks that fit its chemical keys?* If not, then don't eat it, drink it, inject it, snort it, breathe it, or rub it into your skin.

Third Principle of Sports Nutrition
Design your diet and lifestyle so that you avoid, expel or neutralize all chemicals invented by man.

4

PHYSIOLOGICAL DYNAMICS

Every commerce-driven day, hundreds of magazines, newspapers, TV ads and now the internet, bombard bewildered consumers with ads claiming that this or that nutrient will lift your body and your spirits to new heights of health and performance. And hundreds of silly researchers do even sillier short-term experiments, searching for so-called "ergogenic" effects of this or that nutrient. Or worse, they ply unsuspecting subjects with "ancient," "secret" formulas, usually bogus, concocted with anything from Chinese worms to the slime of warty toads.

It boils my blood to see such quackery appearing in learned journals pretending to be nutrition science. To put it plain and simple, *all* short-term human experiments with nutrients done for a few weeks to a few months have nothing, nada, zero, zilch to do with nutrition.

Yes, as we will see ahead you can create short-term ergogenic (performance enhancing) effects with all sorts of substances, especially drugs. That's not nutrition! It's just a temporary accelerated use of bodily resources for which you have to pay the piper down the road.

Nutrition consists of understanding the basic chemistry of the body, and its physiological dynamics of growth, so that you can supply the ancient materials from which it is constructed in the right ratios and amounts and for long enough, to build and repair it optimally in relation to the environmental stresses it confronts. In short, the business of correct nutrition is to build a better body. Unlike the rapid and temporary effects of drugs, or other concoctions, nutrients work slowly. They have to have the time to grow into your structure.

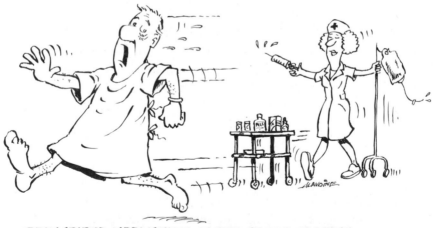

PRESCRIBED MEDICATION IS ONE OF OUR BIGGEST CAUSES OF DISEASE

Waiting On Nature

To build better cells, you have to wait on Nature to eliminate defective and worn out cells. Your skin, the biggest organ of your body is replaced every two weeks. Your whole blood supply is replaced every three months. Most of the cells in your muscles are replaced every six months. In a year even the DNA of your genes is replaced. All of it grows silently and inexorably out of what you eat, drink and breathe.

The body also changes its response to improved nutrition. Throughout at least one year, absorption and use of supplementary nutrients rises dramatically, as the body adapts its enzyme production and other mechanisms to take advantage of the enriched nutrient mix. Whenever anyone quotes you a standard for nutrition, ask for the studies and their duration from which the standard was derived. If they don't know, reject them as charlatans. If they do know, and the studies ran for less than a year, *don't believe them*.

Waiting for the growth is tough. In our instant mashed potato society, everyone is looking for a quick fix. For athletic excellence there's no such animal, nor will there ever be. But the power of Nature to translate the right nutrition and training into a new body is well worth the wait. Touring professional golfer Richard Hall came to me in 1999 to gain some strength. In 18 months he has put on 26 lbs of muscle, does push-ups with 100 lbs of plates on his back, and is aiming to out-drive Tiger Woods.

It's simple. If you consume mostly garbage, you will gradually grow a garbage body, no matter how many "miracle" ergogenic concoctions you take. But, if you consume the best of the structural materials that your body needs, over a long period, you give it the freedom to express its genetic heritage and grow like a god.

Look at it this way. Without correct nutrition and training, the human body is like a neglected houseplant, dull, droopy, no sparkle. Given the right plant food, water, fresh air, light and TLC, the plant will perk up a bit. But you have to wait on Nature for the old defective leaves and stems to die off, and new ones to grow, to see the real expression of its genetic makeup. In six months the plant is sleek with budknots and the leap of life. With a couple of years of continuous care it will grow to magnificence.

Fourth Principle of Sports Nutrition

Nutritional effects have to wait on physiological dynamics. Formulate a precise nutrition and training plan, and arrange your lifestyle so that you enjoy it and can stick to it for at least two years.

5

SOME FOLK HAVE FAT FEET

Stores sell thousands of one-size-fits-all sports nutrition supplements, as if they are right for everyone. No way! Look around. Some folk have fat feet, others have skinny feet, long feet, short feet, high feet, flat feet. The range of physiological variations in feet is such that one-size-fits-all shoes would hardly fit anyone. You are at least as genetically individual as your feet, and require a nutrition program tailored to that individuality.

Maybe you put on bodyfat easily. If so, you need different nutrition and training than folk who eat the refrigerator and stay skinny as a rail. You need higher protein, lower glycemic-index carbohydrates, and lower fat than they do. You need more of the nutrients that support your insulin metabolism, such as chromium, and also more of the nutrients that shift your metabolism towards the glucagon end of the insulin-glucagon axis, such as omega-3 essential fats.

Or maybe you are one of those athletes who suffer acid stomach, while your buddy's nickname is "Ironguts." You need better low-acid nutrition and more acid-buffering foods and supplements than he does. He can drink orange juice by the liter, whereas you should avoid it like the plague.

Perhaps you are a hard-gainer, someone who has great difficulty developing muscle and strength. You need more nutrients and training that reduce muscle catabolism, increase nitrogen retention and maximize your anabolic drive. You also need to schedule your nutrition and training to fit with your circadian rhythms, to take advantage of points on the daily cycle during which the body better retains nitrogen.

Individual athletes also vary widely in nutrient needs because of body size, bodyweight, training intensity, medication, particular sport and dozens of other factors. Tiny Naoko Takahashi, gold medallist in the 2000 Olympic marathon has very different nutrition needs than men's hundred-meter champion Maurice Greene. And elite athletes need a lot more concentrated nutrition than weekend warriors who can train only an hour a day.

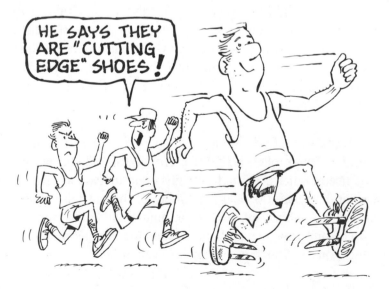

Sports Individuality

Then there are the demands of your sport. If you are a strength athlete, a sprinter or a short anaerobic performance athlete, you need more nutrients and the right training to enhance nitrogen retention, reduce muscle catabolism, increase fast-twitch muscle fiber growth and minimize body fat.

If you are an endurance runner covering 100 miles a week, you will not be concerned about bodyfat because you use it all in training. You will want the right nutrition and training for slow-twitch muscle fiber growth and increased VO$_2$ max. You will also need a specific Colgan Power Program and Nutrition to develop maximum strength per pound of lean mass. Because of your vastly increased oxygen consumption, you should also arrange your lifestyle so that you run in unpolluted air so as to reduce free radical damage. You also need a high intake of antioxidants to offset the enormous oxidation damage caused by long endurance training.

Throughout this book we cover hundreds of such individual differences, so you can **design your nutrition and training to fit your genetic individuality and your sport, at least as well as the right shoes fit your feet.**

Fifth Principle of Sports Nutrition

Design your nutrition and training to suit your genetic individuality and the particular demands of your sport.

"Those who tell you that your nutrition needs are the same as the next man's, have no appreciation of the scale of genetic individuality. Without such as appreciation, they have no understanding of the nutrition needs of anyone."

- Michael Colgan
Sports Nutrition Lecture Series, 2001

6

SEVEN STEPS TO GLORY

School children are still being wrongly taught that good nutrition is a simple matter of eating a balanced diet. Any time you see or hear the term "balanced diet" do not believe *anything* that the person uttering it has to say.

Why am I so sure that they are either lying or ignorant? Let me tell you. For more than 50 years, up to the early 1990's, a balanced diet meant eating three square meals a day from the Four Food Groups, meats, dairy foods, grains, and fruits and vegetables. This official "balanced diet" was conceived by commercial interests primarily as a ploy to sell high-fat meats and dairy foods. It had nothing to do with human health. On the contrary, because of the high-fat load imposed on the American population, the Four Food Groups caused a great deal of our current epidemics of cardiovascular disease and cancer.[1,2]

Dr. Denis Burkitt among many others amply documented the increases in disease and degradation caused directly by following the Four Food Groups.[2] But the commercial greed behind the scam was too powerful. Thousands of text books were written and tens of thousands of well meaning, though not very intelligent, teachers and dieticians were trained to spread this false gospel, until it became accepted public knowledge. If you think it incredible that the teachers and the public could be so easily fooled, remember it is only 100 years ago that most folk believed in sorcery and church leaders condemned unfortunate women as witches.

It took 20 years, from 1970-1990 of continuing objection to the Four Food Groups by thousands of scientists, including us at the Colgan Institute, to finally beat the food lobbies and have the scam thrown out. In 1992 the US Department of Agriculture reluctantly introduced the Eating Right Pyramid.[3] It wasn't what scientists had asked for, but was a compromise with the food lobbies, especially the cereal lobby. But at least it was going in the right direction. Shown here in Figure 1, the pyramid reduces the fat content of the diet and apportions food somewhat in relation to its requirements by the human body.

The big remaining problem is the bread, cereal, rice and pasta group. The Pyramid advises you to eat twice as much of this category every day as any other. Both the evolutionary history of humans, and the new science of nutrition, show clearly that the vegetable and fruit groups should constitute the largest part of the diet at the base of the pyramid.

Also, the Pyramid makes no distinction between whole grains and the poor excuse for them presented in most cereal goods, as white flour or so-called "enriched" flour. In fact, most breads and cereals labeled "whole grain" in the United States are still made primarily from white or enriched flour. These edibles are about as related to the foods we evolved on, as that ghastly glop called "fruit leather" is to real fruit. Nevertheless, tens of thousands of well-meaning teachers are now imparting this new false gospel of a balanced diet to their students. If your goal is athletic excellence, leave it to the wannabes.

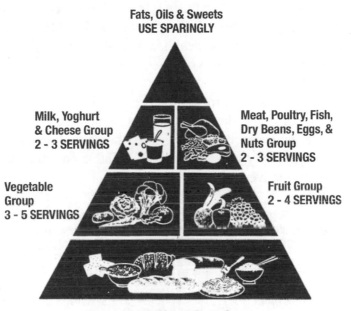

Fats, Oils & Sweets
USE SPARINGLY

Milk, Yoghurt
& Cheese Group
2 - 3 SERVINGS

Meat, Poultry, Fish,
Dry Beans, Eggs, &
Nuts Group
2 - 3 SERVINGS

Vegetable
Group
3 - 5 SERVINGS

Fruit Group
2 - 4 SERVINGS

Bread, Cereal, Rice, & Pasta Group
6 - 11 SERVINGS

Figure 1:
Eating Right Pyramid. Re-drawn from USDA Publication
No. 252, MD:USDA, 1992

Balance and Completeness

The First Principle of sports nutrition, covered in Chapter 1, is that you eat only those ancient nutrients upon which the human body evolved. The Second Principle, covered in Chapter 2, is that you design your diet so that you receive a complete and proportionate mix of these nutrients every day. To assist you to follow these principles, we developed a food pyramid that more accurately reflects human evolutionary heritage and bodily needs.

Shown in Figure 2, the Food Pyramid For Athletes reverses the position of grains and fruits and vegetables. Ancient man lived primarily by foraging for wild edibles.[2] In his book **The Power Of Superfoods**, my friend Sam Graci provides a delightful account of this history and the effects on health.[4] Vegetables and fruits therefore should form the solid base of your diet.

Our ancestors did not process foods either. They ate grains whole including the germ and the essential fiber, which are removed from modern white and enriched flours. So our pyramid stresses whole grains, and organically grown, to mimic as far as possible the grains upon which we evolved.

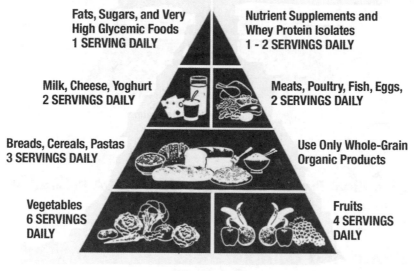

Fats, Sugars, and Very High Glycemic Foods
1 SERVING DAILY

Nutrient Supplements and Whey Protein Isolates
1 - 2 SERVINGS DAILY

Milk, Cheese, Yoghurt
2 SERVINGS DAILY

Meats, Poultry, Fish, Eggs,
2 SERVINGS DAILY

Breads, Cereals, Pastas
3 SERVINGS DAILY

Use Only Whole-Grain Organic Products

Vegetables
6 SERVINGS
DAILY

Fruits
4 SERVINGS
DAILY

Figure 2:
Colgan Institute Food Pyramid for Athletes

The Athletes' Pyramid consists of 20 servings daily. The first 10 at the base, that is, 50% of your diet, should consist of fruits and vegetables, unprocessed of course, and organically grown if you can get them. The second layer of the Athletes' Pyramid, that is, 20% of your diet, consists of 4 servings of whole grains, again organically grown and minimally processed. The third layer of 4 servings, that is, 20% of your diet, consists of dairy foods, eggs, meats and fish. The top layer consists of one serving of fats and sugars, excepting essential fats, that is, 5% of your diet.

The top layer also includes 1-2 servings of whey protein isolates, either ion-exchange or cross-flow membrane extracted, plus 1-2 servings of multi mineral/vitamin and adjunctive nutrient supplements. These are included because of the degradation of our food supply discussed in previous chapters, and well documented in numerous other writings.[1,5,6]

Admittedly, inclusion of pills and extracted whey proteins is a compromise, though a necessary one forced upon us by modern life, if we are to get anywhere near to matching the amounts and the complete range of essential nutrients found in ancient foods. The necessity of the whey protein is well documented in Volume 2. The Food Pyramid for Athletes forms the Sixth Principle of Sports Nutrition:

Sixth Principle of Sports Nutrition
Make the Food Pyramid for Athletes the basis of your nutrition.

The Glycemic Index

First developed by Dr. David Jenkins in 1971, to assist diabetics to stabilize their blood sugar, the Glycemic Index measures the magnitude of the blood sugar response to different foods. Pure glucose, one of the worst foods, is taken as the standard, representing a 100% blood sugar spike.

I should mention however, that some lists use white bread as the 100% mark, which makes glucose 138-142, depending on whose standard you take. These variations confuse a lot of people. The pure glucose standard is more accurate, because the blood sugar spike to white bread varies considerably depending on the flour used to make it, baking methods, the age of the bread and numerous other factors. So here we will stick to the glucose standard used with diabetics.

It is not only diabetics who should strive to maintain blood sugar stability. This strategy applies to all of us if we want optimal health. The science is well documented in Volume 2. Suffice to say here that eating a low-glycemic diet:

1. Enables your body to gradually learn to produce energy more easily from its structure, and to be much less dependent on the food in your gut.
2. Minimizes the hypoglycemic effect of sudden intense exercise.
3. Increases the free fatty acids in the bloodstream, thereby enabling you to spare muscle glycogen during exercise.
4. Reduces your appetite for quick sugars and carbohydrates that spike blood sugar.
5. Maintains insulin sensitivity and efficiency.
6. Keeps blood stable, including during exercise. Blood sugar stability is essential for growth of muscle and strength and for the even flow of energy.[5,7-10]

The evidence that a low-glycemic diet gradually changes your body towards optimum performance, is now so strong that I have made it the Seventh Principle of Sports Nutrition:

Seventh Principle of Sports Nutrition
Eat a low-glycemic diet.

To assist you to eat low-glycemic foods, Tables 3 and 4 show a short list of common foods extracted from the Colgan Institute Glycemic database. Of necessity, many of the broad categories, such as whole-wheat bread are given an average glycemic index number derived from the varying scores of numerous different brands.

Nevertheless the numbers are sufficiently accurate to plan a good diet.

Avoid the high-glycemic list and eat heartily from the low-glycemic list. Meats, fish, eggs, and whey protein isolates are not included because they are all low-glycemic. When eaten together with high-glycemic foods, they also have the added advantage of lowering the overall glycemic index of the meal.

Table 3: High-glycemic Foods

High-glycemic Foods: 60-100%
Spike Blood Sugar and Insulin: AVOID these Foods

BREADS		Grapenut flakes	80	FRUITS	
Dark rye	76	Total	76	Dates	99
White wheat	72	Corn Bran	75	Watermelon	72
Wholewheat	69	Cheerios	74	Cantaloupe	65
Cornmeal	68	Puffed wheat	74	Pineapple	65
BAKED GOODS		Shredded wheat	69	Apricots, canned	64
Rice cakes	94	Grapenuts	67	VEGETABLES	
Waffle	76	Life	66	Instant potato	84
Doughnut	76	Cream of wheat	66	Baked potato	83
Kaiser roll	73	Instant Oatmeal	66	Mashed potato	75
Bagel	72	Nutrigrain	66	Pumpkin	75
Croissant	67	Swiss Museli	60	Carrots	74
Angel food cake	67	PASTAS		Beets	64
CEREALS		Brown rice pasta	92	LEGUMES	
Puffed rice	90	Gnocchi	68	None	
Rice Chex	89	GRAINS		BEVERAGES	
Crispix	87	Rice, instant	92	Canned juice nectars	72
Corn Chex	83	Rice, white	92	Sodas	72
Cornflakes	83	Millet	75	SNACKS	
Rice Crispies	82	Cornmeal	68	Dates	99
Team	82	Couscous	65	Mini rice cakes	90

High-glycemic Foods: 60-100%
(cont'd)

Graham crackers	74	Raisins	64	**SUGARS**	
Corn chips	73	**SWEETS**		Glucose	100
Potato chips	62	Jelly beans	80	Honey	68
Wheat crackers	67	Skittles	70	Sucrose	65
Shortbread	64	Lifesavers	70		

Table 4: Low-glycemic Foods

Low-glycemic Foods: Below 60%
Help maintain blood sugar & insulin stability:
Eat these Foods

BREADS		**PASTAS**		Orange	43
Pita	57	Linguine, durum	50	Peach	42
Wholewheat pita	55	Macaroni	46	Apple	36
Whole rye	52	Spaghetti	41	Pear	36
Pumpernickel	49	Vermicelli	35	Strawberry	32
BAKED GOODS		**GRAINS**		Plum	24
Danish	59	Brown rice	57	Grapefruit	23
Bran muffin	59	Buckwheat	54	Cherries	22
Banana cake	50	Bulgur	48	**VEGETABLES**	
Sponge cake	48	Whole rye	34	Sweet Potato	54
CEREALS		Barley	23	Yams	51
Bran Chex	58	**FRUITS**		Green peas	48
Special K	54	Papaya	58	Tomatoes	38
Oatmeal, slow cooked,		Banana	58	Squash	29
old-fashioned	52	Mango	55	Cucumber	24
All Bran	44	Kiwi	52	Broccoli, cauliflower,	
Rice Bran	20	Grapes	46	cabbage, lettuce very low	

Low-glycemic Foods: Below 60%
(cont'd)

Peppers, onions, radishes very low		Soy beans	18	Popcorn	55
LEGUMES		**BEVERAGES**		Oatmeal cookies	55
Baked beans	48	Orange juice	57	Digestive cookies	54
Pinto beans	42	Pineapple juice	46	Peanuts	18
Brown beans	39	Grapefruit juice	40	Soybeans	18
Navy beans	38	Skim milk	32	**SWEETS**	
Butter beans	32	Milk	28	Ice cream	59
Split peas	32	Agave juice	15	Chocolate	50
Chickpeas	32	Tea	0	Peanut M & M's	35
Green beans	30	Coffee	0	**SUGARS**	
Lentils	30	Water	0	Lactose	46
Kidney beans	27	**SNACKS**		Fructose	23
		Figs	59		

To summarize the seven first steps to glory:

1. Take into your body only those ancient nutrients upon which humankind evolved.
2. Design your diet so that you receive a complete and proportionate mix of all the nutrients every day.
3. Avoid, expel or neutralize all chemicals invented by man.
4. To effect a lasting benefit, stick to your nutrition plan for at least two years, and preferably indefinitely.
5. Design your nutrition and training to suit your genetic individuality and the particular demands of your sport.
6. Make the Food Pyramid For Athletes the base of your nutrition.
7. Eat a low-glycemic diet.

Now you are ready to consider the minerals, vitamins, adjunctive nutrients and anti-oxidants that will speed your progress.

"Do not open the door of your sensibilities unless you are ready, for you will no longer know peace until you pass through the portal."

- Michael Colgan
Program Your Mind Lecture Series, 2001

7

MINERAL MAKEOVER

If someone calls you a "gasbag", they are nearer the truth than most people think. Three quarters of you (and me) is made from two gaseous elements, **oxygen** (65%) and **hydrogen** (10%). We are all mainly hot hair. Add the elements **carbon** (18.5%) and **nitrogen** (3%) and you have over 95% of the human body.

You get plenty of oxygen and hydrogen from air and water, and carbon and nitrogen from proteins, carbohydrates and essential fats, all covered in Volume 2 of this series. But, today, most of these sources are variously polluted and interfered with by man. Unless you get them right first, then none of the other nutrients can work properly. That's why smart athletes live in unpolluted air, drink pure water, and eat uncontaminated proteins and unprocessed carbohydrates and essential fats.

Once you get the big bits right, next as a percentage of body structure come **calcium** (1.2%), **phosphorus** (1.0%), **potassium** (0.4%), **sulfur** (0.3%), **chloride** (0.2%), **sodium** (0.2%) and **magnesium** (0.1%). These elements are very unevenly distributed in foods and varyingly bioavailable in different foods, so you need exactly the right diet, including supplementation in order to obtain correct amounts.

Sulfur is a special case. It used to be so well supplied in plant and animal foods that it was ignored in books and recommendations on nutrition. But soil degradation and food processing have reduced the sulfur content of food to such an extent that champion livestock, such as racehorses, are now routinely supplemented with sulfur to improve their performance. Recent evidence suggests that champion humans, that is athletes, thrive on similar supplementation.

All the other 19 essential minerals are more correctly called **trace elements** because, together with all the vitamins and all other nutrients, they comprise less than 0.1% of your structure. Yet without any one of them you would slowly shrivel up and die. The elemental construction of the human body is laid out in Table 5 ahead.

Some trace elements, nickel, tin and arsenic are essential for animals, and probably essential for humans, but we don't know a lot about them yet in human nutrition, so can't say how much of each is required. For the rest, the following guide is as definitive as the latest science permits.

Note well that mineral elements, including those in gaseous form, make up virtually all your structure and are the primary controllers of virtually all your functions. The other bits and pieces, vitamins and adjunctive nutrients have much lesser functions in comparison. You function primarily by way of gases and a little bit of dirt. All the so-called ergogenic concoctions such as tribulus, creatine, yohimbe, ephedrine, ginseng, CLA, OKG, HMB, KIC and uncle Tom Covvly and all, have hardly any function. Nature spent millions of years designing the human system to work best on a precise combination of the elements used to make it. Unless you get these right first, anything else you put into your body is a waste of time and money. It's like trying to improve the performance of my Porsche by fine-tuning the gas mixture with additives, when the fuel tank is full of crud.

We will consider each mineral under six criteria:

- **Major functions**

- **Food sources**

- **Are athletes deficient?**

- **How to measure status**

- **How much do athletes need?**

- **Toxicity**

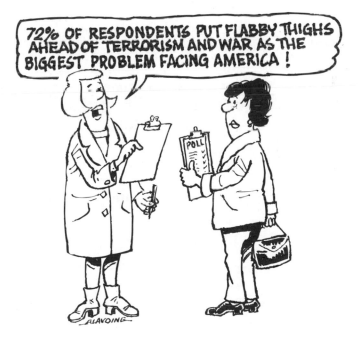

Table 5:
Composition of the Human Body

Gaseous Elements		
Oxygen		65 %
Hydrogen		10 %
Nitrogen		3 %
	Total	78 %
Mineral Elements		
Carbon		18.5 %
Calcium		1.2 %
Phosphorus		1.0 %
Potassium		0.4 %
Sulfur		0.3 %
Sodium		0.2 %
Chloride		0.2 %
Magnesium		0.1 %
	Total	99.9 %
Trace Elements and all Other Nutrients		0.1%
	Total	100%

8

CALCIUM

About 99% of your 3 lbs (1.4 kg) or so of calcium is built into your bones. The remaining 1% circulates around, involved in myriad functions from conduction of nerve impulses to contraction of muscles. To stay alive, your circulating calcium has to remain within narrow limits. Too much and it calcifies your tissue into stone: too little and it cannibalizes your skeleton to make up the deficit.

Calcium deficienty is far more common than excess. Calcium intake in America averages only 740 mg per day,[1] way below the RDI of 1000-1200 mg. Two women in every three aged between 18 and 35 get insufficient calcium.[2] Adolescents are also grossly deficient.[3] Multiple studies show that, despite the milky upper lip of sports celebrities on TV, many athletes, especially females, are way short on calcium.[4-6]

Good food sources of calcium are dairy products and leafy greens, but you excrete about two-thirds of it. A large glass of milk may contain 500 mg of elemental calcium, but only about 150 mg gets absorbed.[7] **Oxalates** in food such as chocolate, cocoa, coffee, spinach and rhubarb, and **phytates** in grains, also bind calcium and make it unavailable to the body. Chocolate milk provides children with very little calcium. In a good mixed diet, calcium is more difficult to get than most people think.

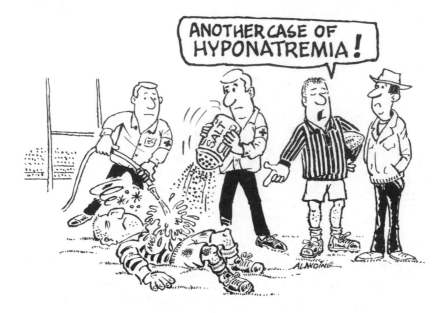

Calcium, Hormones, Muscle and Bone

I want to show you that athletes require a great deal more calcium than the RDI, and that most are not getting it. We know that it takes at least 1000 mg of calcium per day (plus a lot of other nutrients) to maintain normal bone density in sedentary folk.[8] But exercise uses a lot more calcium,[9] especially in combination with high protein diets.[10] We don't know exactly how much. But it's enough to have respected researchers, such as Weaver of Purdue University in Indiana, calling for calcium requirements to be specified in relation to the amount of exercise a person does.[8]

Estimating calcium for athletes is a bit of a detective story, but it's worth the effort. Many researchers have found that the high-volume training that all athletes have to do today if they want to become elite, causes marked declines in steroid hormone levels and serious loss of bone. These losses occur in both in both male and female athletes.[11-13]

Recent studies show there are also detrimental changes in the hypo-thalamus and pituitary in the brain, and in the adrenal glands and sex organs.[14-16]

This bone and muscle loss syndrome from intense exercise is most obvious in female athletes. It is often included in **the female athlete triad** of anorexia, amenorrhea and osteoporosis covered in chapters ahead, and is attributed to estrogen loss and to nutrient intakes well below the RDI.[14-16] Big mistake! We know now that is not the problem.

We have found numerous female athletes who eat very well, and supplement regularly with all nutrients including calcium, to well above the RDI, who still exhibit amenorrhea and bone loss. As each competitive season progresses, these women also lose substantial muscle and strength and report reduced libido. Studies show clearly, however, that estrogen is hardly at all related to muscle. Amenorrheic women given estrogen replacement plus weight training, do not gain more strength than amenorrheic women given weight training alone.[15,17] So there's a lot more to it than estrogen loss.

Well-fed and supplemented males under high volume training also show muscle loss, bone loss, and hypothalamic-pituitary distur-bances which reduce libido and sperm count.[18-20] Their estrogen lev-els, however, are unaffected. Instead they show testosterone decline.

So here's the puzzle. Females lose estrogen which might account for their amenorrhea and bone loss, but not for their muscle loss. Males lose testosterone which might account for their muscle loss and reduced libido, but not for their bone loss. What is the missing factor that ties it all together? From a variety of clues, we reasoned that it might be a greatly increased demand for calcium that is caused by exercise.

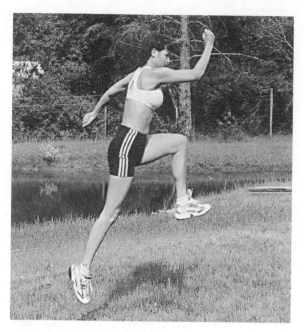

Karen Reynolds showing great form training at the Colgan Institute facility on Saltspring Island in British Columbia.

Mineral Nutrition Is Nature's Key

Calcium is the main mineral in bone, and moderate exercise is known to increase bone calcium and bone strength.[21] But the data in the above studies show bone loss, which means that calcium is being taken from bone for use in exercise. So part of the answer has to involve calcium malnutrition.

This reasoning runs counter to the prevailing belief that, even with exercise, losses of calcium in urine and sweat are a maximum of about 150 mg per day.[22,23] How could more calcium do any good? To find out, we supplemented well-fed but amenorrheic female athletes with increased doses of calcium (2000 mg) plus other nutrients intimately involved in bone: magnesium, phosphorus, fluoride, silicon, zinc, copper, boron, manganese, vitamin D, and vitamin K.[1] Over six months, we got spectacular results, both in increased bone density and muscle gain.

But we had only our hunch and these cases to go on, so could not broadcast the results as scientific evidence. Then along came controlled research to support us. In a representative study, Robert Kiesges and colleagues at the University of Memphis found that an intense 2–hour training session can cause sweat losses of 400 mg of calcium in male athletes.[24] Two of those sessions per day, which is common in many sports, and you need an extra 800 mg of calcium to combat calcium loss in sweat alone.

With absorption of calcium from food and supplements being only about 33%[1,7] to get 800 mg into the bloodstream, you would need to eat an extra 2400 mg of calcium. Add that to the 1000 mg intake required for body maintenance in sedentary life, and you get a whopping 3400 mg total calcium intake per day. Few athletes get anywhere near that much.

Prompted by their sweat loss data, Kiesges and colleagues followed a Division 1-A men's basketball team for a year of training and competition. They found substantial bone loss and negligible gain in muscle. Throughout the next year they gave the athletes 1000-1800 mg calcium per day plus calcium-rich drinks, depending on the degree of bone loss the previous year. The athletes were ingesting 1600-2400 mg calcium in addition to what was in their diet. Over the season they steadily gained bone mass. And by the end of it they had also gained an average of 2 kg (4.4 lbs) of muscle.[24]

Adding the new research to our own case studies, we are now convinced that athletes in intense training need supplementary calcium of 1000-2000 mg per day, plus greater amounts of the other nutrients involved in bone that are noted above. Each of these this chapters ahead. This simple nutritional intervention may offset a great deal of illness, bone loss, muscle loss, stress fractures and misery that currently besets both male and female athletes.

Don't believe any nig nog who tells you that athletes have adequate calcium status without these amounts. Calcium status of athletes is very difficult to measure. The usual measure on a blood screen, **serum calcium** is next to useless because your body has tight controls which keep blood calcium within a narrow range unless you have serious illness. Also, blood levels give no clue to calcium status of soft tissues or bones. Based on a combination of factors including bone density and muscle gain, we use daily supplements of 1000 – 2000 mg of calcium as carbonate and citrate with athletes. Don't pop calcium pills willy-nilly, however. Above 2,500 mg per day, calcium can cause kidney stones and disrupt the balance of iron and zinc.[1,25] Toxicity of our range – nil.

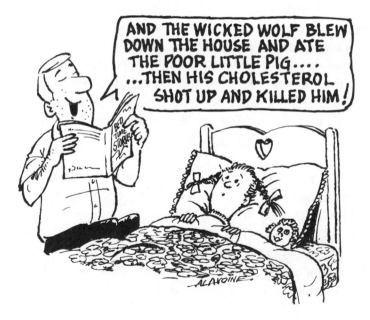

9

PHOSPHORUS

About 85% of the **phosphorus** in your body is part of your bones. The other 15% is essential for virtually every bodily function.[1] Adenosine triphosphate (ATP), your basic energy compound, consists of one molecule of adenosine bonded to three molecules of phosphate. One of these phosphate molecules is used up as ATP is converted to energy. The ATP is then regenerated by a phosphate molecule taken from creatine phosphate stored in the muscle.

Your body also uses phosphorus mixed with vitamin B_6 as **pyridoxal phosphate** to make new muscle glycogen. Phosphorus is again essential to convert the glycogen to energy because it forms part of the enzyme **phosphofructokinase**, the rate-limiting step in glycogen use.[2] It also forms part of **2-3-diphosphoglycerate** which enables the hemoglobin of red blood cells to unload oxygen into muscle cells. And, when the muscle has contracted, phosphorus also acts as an **alkaline buffer** to reduce acidity. Without sufficient phosphorus you couldn't move a muscle.

Phosphorus occurs widely in foods and is also added to many foods during processing. Best sources in order of phosphorus content

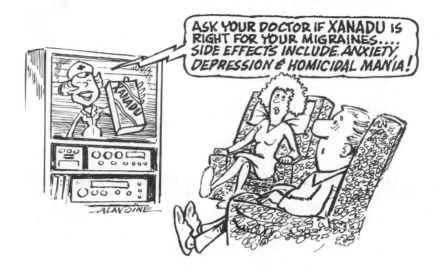

are meats, fish, dairy products and whole grains. Average intake in the US is about 1500 mg per day for males and 1000 mg/day for females,[1] much higher than the intake of calcium, and well above the RDA for phosphorus of 800 mg per day.

Aluminum in consumer goods binds phosphorus preventing absorption. But no serious athlete should use products containing the poison metal aluminum anyway, including toothpastes, antacids, deodorants and hair products. Look for words "alumina," "alum" and words beginning with "alum" and leave those products on the shelf.

Phosphorus For Athletes

Because they use 12-20 times the energy of sedentary folk, athletes need a lot more phosphorus. We also know this, because we and other researchers have found blood phosphorus levels of non-supplemented trained athletes (which appear in the blood as phosphates) to be 1.5 -1.9 nmol/l, well above the range for the general public of 0.75-1.35 nmol/l.[3]

Even with such high resting blood levels, endurance athletes may show very low levels of phosphate after long exercise, indicating heavy phosphate use. So their phosphorus intake may not be optimal.[4,5]

Research during the early '90s on phosphate loading of athletes supports this idea. Studies from a wide range of laboratories show that acute doses of 4.0 grams of phosphate per day have three distinct effects. First, they reduce muscle acidity.[6,7] Second, they increase production of glycogen for fuel.[2] Third, they raise levels of 2-3-diphosphoglycerate the enzyme that unloads oxygen from hemoglo bin into muscle.[8,9]

These studies, called "phosphate loading," also significantly improved performance. Robert Cade and his group at the University of Florida, for example, reported increases in VO2 max of 6-12% and increases in time to exhaustion on the treadmill of 3-9 minutes.[9] Ian Stewart and colleagues at the Tasmanian Institute of Technology in Australia found increases of 11% in VO2 max, and a huge 20% increase in time to exhaustion.[8] Richard Krieder and colleagues at Old Dominion University in Virginia reported an increase in maximal power output of 17%. That's big![10]

Despite these and similar studies, over the last five years, phosphate loading has fallen out of favor with athletes. As we have observed, use of high doses of sodium phosphate (the usual supplement form) frequently causes intestinal discomfort, gas, nausea and other nasties. Also, phosphate loading may work once or twice, but then fades as your body learns to neutralize the non-physiological and therefore toxic effects. So, when you add in the side-effects, the net effect in real-life sports competition may be performance decline. Leave it for the wannabees.

Large, acute doses of phosphate also interfere with calcium metabolism causing body loss of calcium.[1] As occurs with any nutri-ent, dumping a big bolus of the stuff into that biochemical mix that you call "me" leads to a net loss of function, if not immediately then somewhere down the road.

Always consider nutrients as building blocks. You put in the right amounts every day, to gradually build your body to a steady state of action potential which enables it to express its genetic design to the max. Anything else, any overdose of nutrients to create an ergogenic boost, is a temporary drug-like effect which squanders the body's resources and inevitably comes back to bite you.

No reliable test of phosphorus status exists for athletes. Because of hemolysis of red cells caused by training, and because of the common practice of phosphorus supplementation, the usual measure, **serum phosphorus** is often falsely elevated.

Regular small supplemental amounts of phosphate over long periods have no side-effects, and may be correcting a deficit to raise phosphate levels to what is more appropriate for athletes. At the Colgan Institute, we now use supplements of 300-1000 mg of phosphorus as **potassium phosphate**. These supplements raise blood phosphorus levels, so we have formulated an athlete normal range for blood phosphate of 1.20 – 1.80 nmol/l. Toxicity of our supplement range – nil.

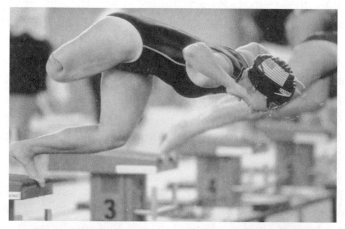

Determination in every muscle of this athlete.

10

POTASSIUM

Your body has three main electrolytes responsible for the flow of electromagnetic energy: **potassium, sodium** and **chloride**. Potassium is the most important. It is called a **cation** because it carries a positive electrical charge. Potassium interacts with the other main cation, sodium, and the **anion** chloride (negatively charged) to enable your nerves to conduct the electrochemical impulses that make you a living being.

All creatures including humans evolved on a high potassium/low sodium diet, because that was the proportion of these minerals, naturally occurring in our ancient environment. So the ideal amount of potassium in your diet should reflect the amount in the foods of our ancient environment. The same foods today, freshly harvested, and unprocessed, are still high in potassium and low in sodium. Even the flesh of sea fish such as salmon and tuna, though they live in an environment with twenty times more sodium than potassium, contain five times more potassium than sodium. Overall, the fresh foods that form a good diet, contain seven times more potassium than sodium. Seven to one is the ratio of Nature's design upon which your body functions best.

In one of the many crimes against human health in the 20th century, food processors reversed this ratio by adding salt to everything. Canned tuna today contains 3-4 times more sodium than potassium. Wholewheat breads contain 5-6 times more sodium than potassium.[1] Overall, the average American diet now contains twice as much sodium as potassium.[2] If you want optimal performance, ***don't eat it!***

Average daily potassium intake in America is about 2.5 grams, much below the recommended amount of 3.5 grams.[2] And a lot of that deficient amount of potassium is promptly excreted, because high fat levels in the average diet block potassium absorption.[2] Some misguided physicians and dieticians scream bloody murder against potassium supplements which might bring the total intake up another gram or so. They seem unaware that folk who eat large amounts of vegetables and fruits get 8-11 grams of potassium per day — and the US National Academy of Sciences reports they are a lot healthier for it.[3]

On Nature's time scale, humanity is still very much a work in progress. We may not reach evolutionary maturity for another couple of million years. One problem still to be worked out by natural selection, is the human body's inability to hold onto sufficient potassium. Unlike most other minerals, we leak potassium like a sieve. Even with insufficient potassium and no exercise, your body cannot conserve this mineral.[4] So unless you base your diet on a wide variety of fruits and vegetables every day, you are likely to be short on both potassium and performance.

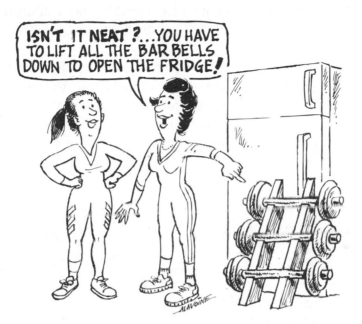

Potassium For Athletes

We know that athletes need more potassium than sedentary folk because one effect of athletic training is a big increase in the potassium content of muscle.[5] Because of potassium use during exercise, and loss of additional potassium in sweat, urine, and hemolysis (bursting of red blood cells), athletes are also in greater danger of potassium deficit than sedentary folk. And the idiotic use of laxatives and diuretics by some athletes trying to "make weight", dumps body potassium faster than spit – a sure way to guarantee potassium deficiency.

Some distance runners have collapsed from potassium deficit.[6] And studies report that low potassium intake is common in wrestlers, gymnasts, track and field athletes, dancers, swimmers and football players.[7] Clearly, they don't eat enough veggies.

Potassium status is commonly measured using **serum potassium,** with 4.5-5.5 mcg/l taken as an acceptable range. It doesn't mean a lot for athletes, because potassium in the blood changes dramatically with exercise, and with the level of carbohydrates in the diet.[8]

The Colgan Institute uses daily supplements of 500 – 2000 mg of potassium as **potassium bicarbonate** with athletes. But mostly we advise at least two meals of a wide variety of vegetables every day, to provide 5-10 grams of potassium. Toxicity – nil. The lowest level at which potassium is reported toxic in an adult is 18 grams per day.[2]

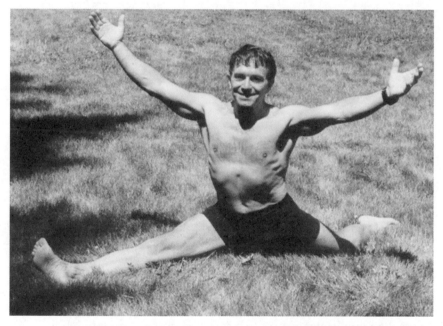

Maintaining flexibility is injury proofing for the body.

SULFUR

You seldom see sulfur even mentioned in human nutrition, and it is rarely included in supplements. There is no discussion of this essential mineral in the RDA Handbook[1] and no official recommendation for its use. Yet your body contains and uses more sulfur than all the 19 trace elements put together, and you cannot make a molecule of sulfur, but must get it from your diet.

Sulfur is essential for everything from use of B-vitamins, to blood coagulation, immune function, antioxidant defenses, and the maintenance of the lining of your heart. But space restricts me to discussing only a couple of systems that are vital to athletes.

Sulfur was left out of human nutrition until recently, because it comes as part of the amino acids of proteins. Eggs and meats are rich sources. Sniff a boiled egg and you smell the sulfur. Most scientists use to believe that the public got plenty of sulfur along with animal protein foods. New research shows this belief is dead wrong. Only some amino acids, such as **cysteine**, contain sulfur, and, if you don't get enough of them, you become sulfur deficient.[2]

Even the slightest sulfur deficiency can whack your performance because it is essential for manufacture of glutathione, one of your main endogenous antioxidants.[2] In a representative study, Lyons and colleagues at Massachusetts Institute of Technology, gave healthy males a diet for 10 days which lacked sulfur amino acids. Compared with a sulfur-rich diet, glutathione synthesis was dramatically reduced.[3] As an athlete in intense training, you are always in free radical overload. You need all the glutathione defenses your body can muster.

Glutathione also functions to maintain immunity. Your T-lymphocytes, discussed in Volume 3 of this series, cannot function without it.[2] Without your T-lymphocyte response to trauma, injury, stress, or bacterial or viral attack, you are prey to every wandering microbe seeking an undefended lunch.

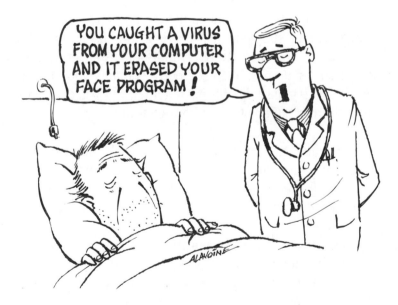

I also want to mention that sulfur is vital to the important **S-ade-nolsylmethionine-homocysteine cycle** discussed in Volume 3 of this series. This cycle is crucial for athletic performance, but is rarely mentioned in books on sports nutrition. New evidence of effects of sulfur deficiency has forced us all to sit up and take more notice.[2,4] If you want to protect your heart, your joints and your brain against the stresses of exercise, S-adenosylmethionine has to function at maximum.[5] Impossible unles syou have sufficient sulfur.

Sulfur For Athletes

All the above considerations prompted the Colgan Institute to begin supplementing athletes with sulfur in 1993. During the ensuing years, we did controlled case studies on athletes, and on horses, showing that sulfur supplementation reduced injury rates and improved joint function in endurance runners, gallopers and jumpers. Results were so compelling that we developed an equine supplement of sulfur containing **methyl-sulfonyl-methane**, (MSM) which is now used by stables world-wide. Now, belatedly, MSM is creeping into human nutrition, too.

There are no reliable measures of human sulfur status. Some researchers at Vernon Young's laboratory at Massachusetts Institute of Technology are just beginning to study it in conjunction with amino acid excretion rates.[6] Despite the lack of a standard, after eight years of our own studies, in conjunction with some new evidence,[2-4] we are pretty confident that sulfur supplementation can protect both joints and immunity. We use daily supplements of 2.0 – 5.0 grams of **methyl-sulfonyl-methane** with athletes. Toxicity – nil

"No amount of fire can drive the engine, except that which is precisely focussed in the pistons."

- Michael Colgan
Program Your Mind Lecture Series, 2001

12

SODIUM AND CHLORIDE

"Canst that which is unsavory be eaten without salt?" One of the 24 references to the benefits of salt in the Bible, Job asked God this rhetorical question in the Old Testament.[1] The Man upstairs may have rained some of the torments he did upon the writers of such piddle, because he knew their careless words would cause even greater suffering to future millions.

Salt is connected by the Good Book to chastity, fellowship, fidelity, fertility and holiness. No surprise that it became a sacred substance that was easy to sell.[2] In early Victorian times when salt became plentiful in the West, Job's question was eventually adopted as an advertising slogan by the world's largest salt company. They became filthy rich, fat and satisfied until hypertension bled their heads off.

Science made possible the manufacturing systems and the transport systems that spread salt liberally all across the world. But, as always, scientific development does not come with instructions as to its beneficial use. The scientific keys that opened the doors of the Industrial Revolution fit equally the locks of Heaven or Hell. The sale of salt in the name of God played right into Satan's hands.

The holy preservative qualities of salt were linked with everything good and wholesome. Salted meats were lauded as better than fresh because they did not rot. And, by using liberal salt, all sorts of offal and fat that was previously discarded, could be made into glorious sausages. Millions of Christians worldwide began gobbling salt like there was no tomorrow, thereby unknowingly thrashing both arteries and kidneys. And the pregnant among them had not an inkling that their offspring would be born with a permanent preference for salt,[3] an addiction that would continue down the generations to pervade our life today.

Blinded by faith, missionaries used salt as a potent enticement to convert, (and addict) African natives. Today, centuries later, a good bit of the high salt preference and rampant hypertension among African Americans[4] may be a direct result of misplaced missionary zeal. For whatever motive, scientific exploitation of the fruits of the Earth always has far-flung consequences.

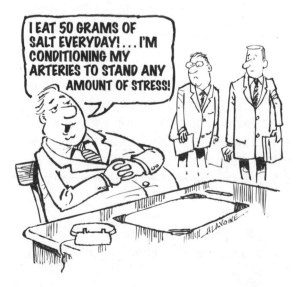

Hypertension Today

By 1900 it became obvious that excess salt was causing widespread hypertension. But, with taste buds and brains dulled by the holy powder, the public and most physicians laughed at Aubard and Beaujard who first documented the connection in 1904. Between then and now incidence of hypertension (systolic 139 + mm Hg, diastolic 89 + mm Hg) has soared to 50 million people in America alone.[5]

Here's a brief sketch of how it happens. Over four million years of evolution humans ate a diet which contained about one gram of sodium chloride per day.[1] At the beginning of the 21st century of "civilization" we eat an average of 9 – 12 grams of salt per day.[6] The human system has not had the evolutionary time to develop any mechanisms to deal with this toxic overload.

Recent research has uncovered some of the ways in which salt does its insidious damage. In folk who eat below 4 gm of salt per day, the body shows a natural **circadian rhythm** of blood pressure. Each night the **sympathetic nervous system** which automatically arouses your organs, slows down, and the **parasympathetic nervous system**, which automatically quiets the body, becomes dominant. This rhythm lowers blood pressure, thus promoting rest and repair of the vascular system and the organs, especially the kidneys.[7]

In folk who eat the American average of about 10 grams grams of salt per day, this circadian rhythm of rejuvenation and sleep is disrupted. Blood pressure either remains high, or gets so low as the body fights the salt, that some hypertensives die of sleep apnea (cessation of breathing). Over years of such misuse, coupled also with the deficient potassium level in Western diets discussed under potassium, the circadian disruption gradually raises blood pressure. The increased pressure then damages the heart, arteries and kidneys, and prematurely ages the salt addict in numerous ways.[6-9]

Comprehensive reviews of the literature to date, just completed by Health Canada and all leading cardiovascular disease authorities, recommend that even healthy people with normal blood pressure:

- Avoid foods high in salt
- Refrain from adding salt at table
- Minimize salt used in cooking
- Increase awareness of salt content of food choices in restaurants.[10]

And some of the world's top researchers on hypertension at Westminster Medical School and St. George's Medical School in London, recently concluded that if we reverted to the low level of dietary salt upon which we evolved, the current epidemic of hypertensive disease would simply disappear.[6,9]

Sodium and Chloride For Athletes

All the above being true, salt is still an essential nutrient. Sodium is a major cation, positively charged electrolyte, and chloride is the main anion, negatively charged electrolyte, in the human body. They work together with potassium to conduct nerve impulses, to control fluid balance, and to regulate certain hormones, plus a host of other jobs.

But most folk need less than one gram of sodium and one gram of chloride in order to function well. Overload is almost always the problem. Athletes are less bothered by the development of hypertension, however, because regular exercise lowers blood pressure even in hypertensives.[11]

The Colgan Institute does not use supplements of sodium or chloride with athletes. The only occasion when these can be useful is in ultradistance endurance events when the athlete has drunk too much water, and is suffering from hyponatremia (salt deficiency). We cover this contingency in Volume 2 of this series.

13

MAGNESIUM

Some 60% of the body's **magnesium** resides in your bones. In conjunction with your basic energy molecules, ATP, the other 40% is essential for all body manufacturing processes, burning of glycogen for fuel, transmission of the genetic code to form new proteins, and the activity of over 300 enzymes.

To accomplish these multiple tasks, your body does everything possible to keep blood magnesium stable between narrow limits. Whenever your diet is short of magnesium the blood steals from your bones to make up the deficit. Once your bones start losing magnesium, they also lose calcium and start breaking up big time. Your kidneys also reabsorb magnesium meticulously and channel it back into the blood, to prevent it being discarded in urine.[1-3]

Best food sources of magnesium are whole grains and legumes, and the chlorophyll in green vegetables. But most of the magnesium in modern food is lost by the removal of the germ and outer layers of grains in making white flour. This processing is done so that the flour has a long shelf life and is easy to cook with, because it is no longer biologically active. Remember this principle: **good food is food that goes bad quickly,** because its biological potential, with which it interacts with your body, also interacts readily with heat, light and air.

Magnesium is only one of the nutrients removed from food by modern processing, but it exemplifies what happened to our mineral nutrition over the 20th century. In just 13 years, from 1976 – 1989 average male magnesium intake in America fell from 354 mg to 329 mg.[3] Current daily intakes are about 320 mg for men and 200 mg for women. These are well below the old RDA of 350 mg and 280 mg respectively. So a lot of Americans are in magnesium deficit.

The picture got worse on 13 August 1997, when the US Institute of Medicine working for the US Academy of Sciences, and for Health Canada, produced a new recommendation for magnesium. This one is called another pedantic name, **estimated average intake** or **EAR**, that is the intake which meets the nutrient needs of half the people in a specific group. For males aged 19-50 the RDA, RDI, DRI, EAR (take your pick) for magnesium is now 400-420 mg per day for males, 310-320 mg for females.[4,5] That puts over 90% of the US and Canadaian population in serious magnesium deficit.

Evidence of the illness caused by low levels of magnesium in American food continues to pour in. A representative study published by the US Centers For Disease Control in Atlanta in 1999, followed a

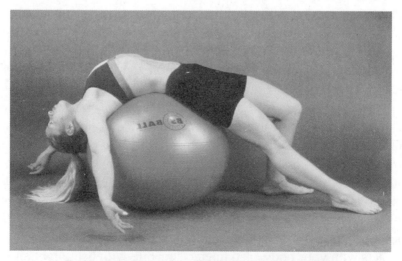

Rest and sleep are where all growth occurs.

national sample of 25,292 adults of all ages, for 19 years. The lower their serum magnesium, the higher the number of deaths from heart disease, and the higher the number of deaths from all causes.[6] Age, sex and other variables made little difference. Low magnesium levels can kill you quick at any age, even in the apparent pink of condition.

Magnesium For Athletes

Because of the greater use of magnesium in energy metabolism, protein synthesis, and the increased losses in magnesium in sweat during exercise, athletes need more magnesium than any other class of people. Yet studies in a wide range of sports including endurance running, triathlon, wrestling, gymnastics and skating, show magnesium intakes below the old RDA.[7-10] Marathon runners also show dramatic declines in serum and urinary magnesium after races, a fair indication of chronic magnesium deficiency.[11] And, from our studies at the Colgan Instututite, we are pretty sure that magnesium deficit is involved in the female athlete syndrome and in male athlete bone loss and stress fractures.

Magnesium status is commonly measured using the **serum magnesium** assay. Below 1.9 mg/dl is taken as a sign of deficit. But the test doesn't tell us diddly about optimal levels. Science has not yet discovered a reliable non-invasive test for magnesium status,[12] and athletes are understandably reluctant to having their organs puréed to set a standard.

The Colgan Institute uses daily supplements of 400-1800 mg of magnesium with athletes, mostly as **magnesium aspartate** which is farily easily absorbed. Many athletes seem well supplied around the middle of this range. For folk with normal kidney function there is no toxicity, because your kidneys will promptly dump any excess.[3]

"The worst moment in life is the moment you lose faith in your dreams. Never let it happen."

- Michael Colgan
Program Your Mind Lecture Series, 2001

14

IRON

Hemoglobin is the red pigment in blood that extracts oxygen from the air in your lungs, and delivers it to your muscles, organs and brain. There the oxygen combines with the energy stored in food to release it for use. Hence the amount of energy you can release, and the level of performance you can reach, largely depend on the amount of hemoglobin in your blood.

In turn production of hemoglobin is largely depends on your body's use of iron. Note well that I said "use of iron" not "iron intake". Although it is an essential nutrient for the formation of hemoglobin, simply eating iron will not do the trick. Another big nutritional error of medicine in the 20th century, was to feed anemic women large doses of iron, especially during pregnancy. This practice, still continued today by old physicians who should have been put out to pasture long since, has caused untold infant deaths, massive maternal illness, and misery all round.[1,2]

The same nonsense was also applied to athletes by medical nignogs, who probably should have been put out to pasture at puberty.[3-5] Alberto Salazar, for example, was the greatest American marathon runner ever. Stricken by runner's anemia in 1984, against my advice he was given large doses of supplemental iron. I predicted then, and published the prediction, that unless Salazar was given a complete synergistic supplement formula containing only a modicum of iron, he would never return to form. Sadly, history has proved me correct.

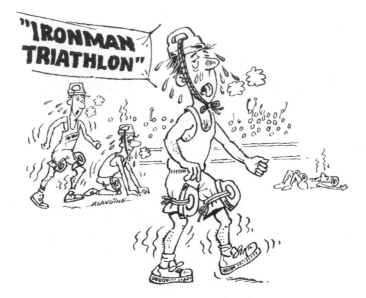

Iron Toxicity

Virtually all animals from bacteria to humans require iron for numerous enzyme functions in order to live and grow. The sole important exception is *Lactobacillus*. Other bacteria all thrive on iron. Nature designed life this way to protect the new-born.

When a human or other mammal baby is born, it has little immune defense. But its gut is sterile and also contains no iron. So the only bacteria that can grow there are *Lactobacillus*. They begin colonizing the gut within minutes after birth, a neat evolutionary device, because these greeblies are essential to digest the mother's milk. Breast milk contains virtually no iron. Harmful bacteria and viruses are kept at bay both by the absence of iron and by multiple immune factors in the milk.

So where do babies get their iron? Many health professionals still seem unaware that babies are born with an iron reserve in their internal tissues and organs, enough to supply them for at least a year.[1,2] Now you know why breast-fed infants are bigger, healthier, smarter and much less subject to infections than bottle-fed.[1,2] Their immune systems are given the chance to develop before the onslaught of aggressive microorganisms.

Bottle-fed babies have no such chance. Bombarded with artificial food containing no immune protectors, and attacked by more microorganisms than you can poke a stick at, they quickly become sickly. Seeing their pallor, or perhaps hoping to thwart Nature, arrogant medicine men often add iron to baby formulas thereby increasing infections, damaging immunity and ensuring that the baby's sickliness proliferates.[1,2]

The same damage happens to athletes given high doses of iron[6], but the effect is harder to spot. Repeated infections and fatigue are often ascribed to overtraining. Typically the athlete is told to back off, but continue the supplement. That creates an even greater iron over-

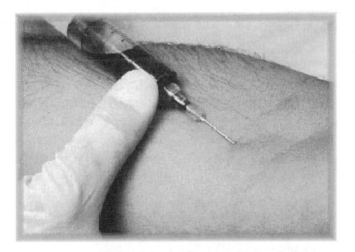

The human body cannot get rid of excess iron. It has to be removed by drawing blood.

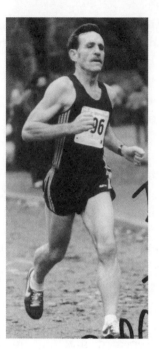

*Masters champion
Bill Misner shows
the form and eyes
closed concentration
that shifts you up
another gear.*

load, thereby worsening the problem. But because the nutritional problems of athletes are seldom properly diagnosed, iron overdoses of 100 mg per day, or more, continue to be recommended.[7]

How Much Iron?

To deal with the important problem of iron nutrition in athletes, first you have to know how much iron athletes use. The 1995 RDI of 18 mg per day is not much help, because it refers only to average sedentary folk. Athletes use, and lose, a lot more iron than that in six different ways: sweat loss, footstrike hemolysis, compression hemolysis, gastrointestinal bleeding, acidosis, and peroxidation of cell membranes by free radicals. I will examine each of these in turn.

On a temperate day, athletes in training sweat about 1.0 – 1.5 liters per hour. That sweat contains about 0.4 – 0.6 mg of iron.[8] Train four hours in a day and you lose 1.6 – 2.4 mg of iron, say an average of 2.0 mg per day.

Footstrike hemolysis, that is destruction of red blood cells caused by the jarring of feet against the ground, occurs in all running athletes.[9,10] Compression hemolysis, that is crushing of red blood cells by intense muscular contraction, also occurs in a wide range of athletes.[11,12] We have found it in weightlifters, and other researchers have found it in cross-country skiers, rowers and swimmers.[11-14] The blood which leaks from both forms of hemolysis is excreted together with the iron it contains. Losses total 0.25 – 0.75 mg per day, say an average of 0.5 mg. Together with sweat loss of iron we are now at about 2.5 mg.

Gastrointestinal bleeding is common in endurance athletes, and acidic gut afflicts about one-third of them. Loss of blood through oxidation damage to cell membranes affects almost all athletes in intense training. Iron loss from these three sources runs about 0.5 - 1.0 mg per day, say an average of 0.75 mg.[15-17]

Added to the other losses, we are now at 3.25 mg of iron lost per day purely as a result of hard exercise. With another 1.0 mg of iron needed for basic functions in males plus an extra 0.5 mg for menstruation loss in females, male athletes in heavy training may need 4.25 mg of iron each day, and females 4.75 mg.

Getting that much iron from food is a tough job. Diets of athletes that we and others have analysed, contain about 6.0 mg of iron per 1000 calories.[18] For a 3,000 calories diet, that's 18 mg of iron per day. But even the best heme iron from meat sources is only 10% absorbed. For the non-heme iron in vegetables, absorption can be as low as 1%.[18] Assuming that the athletes all eat meats, then males need to eat about 42 mg, and females 47 mg of iron every day. That would require an intake of 7,000 calories for males, and 8,000 calories for females. Now you can see why athletes need iron supplements.

Athletes Are Iron Deficient

Only the seriously bulimic can stuff down 8000 calories a day. So it's no surprise that athletes of all stripes are iron deficient. A representative sample of ten of the recent studies from France, Britain, Israel, Scandinavia, Italy, South Africa and the United States show the athletes have low iron intake, low serum ferritin (a reliable measure of the body's iron store), low hemoglobin (the iron containing red pigment in blood) and low hematocrit (the percentage of red blood cells making up the blood).[19-28]

The athletes involved included male and female gymnasts, female discus, hammer and javelin throwers and shotputters, male and female runners, skiers, male boxers, weightlifters and track and field athletes.[19-28] So, anyone who tells you that athletes get enough iron from their diets, is either an ignorant dolt, or has hidden agendas that don't include your welfare.

Diagnosing iron deficiency and poor red blood status in athletes, and correcting them, is so important to performance it deserves a separate chapter. We have spent 20 years devising a successful method. Suffice to say here that the Colgan Institute uses daily supplements of 15 – 40 mg of iron as the most efficiently absorbed form of iron, **iron picolinate**, with athletes. Most are well supplied with 15 – 25 mg. Toxicity of range in properly diagnosed athletes – nil.

15

ZINC

Zinc is essential for all cell growth and forms part of numerous enzymes in every animal and every plant on Earth.[1] The pool of available zinc in the human body is small and rapidly used, so it has to be replaced daily. If you are eating insufficient zinc, your body recognizes the deficit and immediately conserves its supply accordingly by retarding muscle growth, reducing immune activity to a minimum, reducing sexual function, especially in men, and reducing excretion of zinc in body wastes.[1] Not even a sedentary sofa slug can function well on zinc deficiency.

Best food sources of zinc are seafood, meats and eggs. Though it seems readily available in common foods, average intake is rarely sufficient, because absorption of zinc ranges from 40% to a mere 2% depending on the food it is eaten with. Fiber, phytates from grains and vegetables, proteins, and certain minerals in usual mixed meals, all bind zinc and reduce its bioavailability.[2]

Ignoring this wide variation in absorption, almost all studies of zinc status focus on zinc intake alone. In the latest effort, published by the US Centers for Disease Control, only half the US population was judged to get adequate zinc, taking "adequate" to mean an intake of 80% of the RDI of 15 mg per day.[3] With bioavailability so variable, even these supposedly zinc-happy folk, could be absorbing only 0.24

mg of zinc per day. No surprise that impotence is a big worry in America, and Viagra sales are booming.

Also ignored in setting government standards for zinc, are two large avenues of zinc loss. During sex for example, males lose up to 1 mg of zinc per ejaculation.[4] And zinc losses in sweat increase proportionately with exercise.[5] Sweat losses of up to 12 mg of zinc per day are common in athletes.[6]

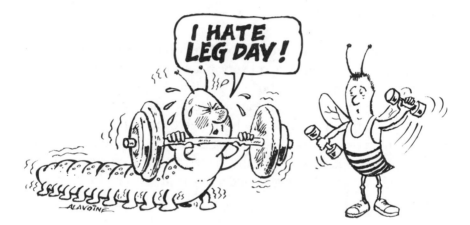

Analysing Zinc Deficiency

Here's a representative case of a fit young Olympic hopeful when he first came to the Colgan Institute with problems of fatigue, repeated infections and performance decline. He was dutifully following the advice of his "sports nutritionist" and eating the RDI of 15 mg of zinc per day, along with other vitamins and minerals, in mixed meals of whole grains, vegetables and proteins. Yet his serum zinc level was way down at 42 mcg/dl, indicating severe zinc deficiency.

Analysing his diet we estimated that zinc absorption was about 20%. So he was absorbing about 3 mg of zinc per day. His training level, which he had increased substantially over the previous six months, combined with the hot environment of San Diego, plus a test we did of his sweat, indicated zinc losses in sweat of 4.5 mg per day. He also reported a highly active sex life of 2-3 ejaculations per day. Knocking two-thirds of that off for wishful thinking, we estimated his seminal zinc loss at 1.0 mg per day. Other losses of zinc in young men in urine and faeces run about 1.5 mg/day.[4] So our subject was absorbing 3 mg of zinc per day and using 7 mg, putting him in severe zinc deficit of 4 mg per day.

"No," objected his nutritionist in her best patronizing voice, "He's just off-color. He's not showing any symptoms of zinc deficiency, such as loss of sexual function, slow healing of wounds, or immune depression." That's the sort of utterance for which the only response is to stuff a raw egg into the offending mouth and tap the jaw smartly – and I wished fervently I had one handy.   With decent supplementation, including 40 mg zinc picolinate per day, we fixed the lad's problem within a few weeks.

This case provides a good illustration of a general principle of sports nutrition that you should get straight, once and for all. Athletes have far superior health and fitness than Mr. and Mrs. Average, from whom the sickness norms used by health professionals are derived. When the average Joe is off-color, has the flu, or an upset gut, is tired, or depressed it's considered just a usual part of life's burden. Those norms do not apply to properly trained and nourished athletes. **Whenever an athlete's health declines to the level of Joe Public's usual health, there's something badly wrong.**

To return to zinc. Respected authorities on mineral nutrition, such as Hambidge at the University of Colorado, agree that science has no reliable biomarkers of mild to moderate zinc deficiency.[7] Science has no standards at all that apply to athletes. We used to refer to studies that measured serum zinc, looking for a level in athletes above 80 mcg/dl. But recent research has confirmed our suspicion, that zinc in the blood does not reflect zinc status in body tissues, except in severe zinc deficiency.[8] When it gets to that stage you are in deep doo-doo.

Zinc For Athletes

Primarily because of advice that they need only the RDI, a lot of athletes are in deep doo-doo over zinc. Low zinc intakes and low blood zinc continue to be reported in many sports including running, track and field, triathlon, wrestling, gymnastics, karate, basketball and skating.[9-16]

Especially in women athletes, a continuing zinc deficiency has consequences more serious than loss of general health and poor sports performance. Multiple studies show that chronic zinc deficiency damages the DNA of your genes, causing what are called **strand breaks** and **oxidative lesions** which raise the risk of cancer later in life into the stratosphere.[17] Health professionals who fail to properly assess an athlete's need for zinc, including the degree of absorption, the maintenance of about 1.5 mg per day, sweat losses of 3 – 12 mg per day and losses during sex, are putting their charges at risk of later fatal disease.

You can get a fair measure of zinc deficiency with a simple serum zinc assay. Acceptable levels for athletes are 80 – 140 mcg/dl. Better measures are complicated and expensive assessments of zinc transport proteins such as albumin.

If you find or suspect zinc deficit, it is easy to fix with supplementation. And there is evidence that supplemental zinc improves strength and muscle metabolism in athletes[18], although these studies could not assess zinc status properly. So we don't know whether the effect was caused by physiological repletion of zinc or a drug-like action. They also used very large doses of zinc, over 100 mg per day.

We advise strongly against such high supplementation. Because of the principle of synergy, large doses of zinc disrupt copper and iron metabolism and other bodily functions.[19]

The Colgan Institute uses daily supplements of 15-50 mg of zinc as **zinc picolinate** with athletes. Most are apparently well supplied at 15-25 mg per day, but extreme endurance sports may require supplementation near the upper end of the range. Toxicity of our range for athletes in regular training – nil.

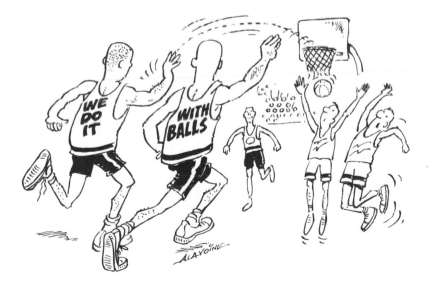

"Empty your mind. Enter competition not angry, not happy, not afraid.
To win, be prepared to die.
You may not succeed in either but you will learn to compete with spirit."

- Michael Colgan
Program Your Mind Lecture Series, 2001

16

COPPER

Copper is involved in so many chemical interactions in the body, I can mention only a few that are pertinent for athletes. It is essential for oxygen use, for the energy cycle, for formation of hemoglobin, and for your immune system to react against stress. It is also used in brain, heart and lung function and in formation of neurotransmitters in nerves. Together with zinc, it forms the vital endogenous antioxidant **copper/zinc superoxide dismutase**, the only potent defense you have against the superoxide **free radical** (02-) discussed in Chapter 49, Antioxidant Armor.[1,2]

Best sources of copper are oysters and beef liver, sunflower seeds, nuts, potatoes and beans. But amounts are highly variable depending on the level of copper in the growing environment.

Copper is a highly reactive metal that changes character very easily. Add a little zinc and it becomes brass. Add a smidgeon of tin and it becomes bronze. Alchemists spent centuries trying to turn copper into gold, but the trick, which modern science can now do easily, forever eluded them.

How Much Copper?

Copper is a similar chameleon in the human body. Too little copper in your mix and you can't even color yourself. Hair goes white and falls out, skin loses its pigment, blood goes blue. Worse, your skeleton disintegrates, and nerves and brain lose their myelin insulation and fuse. You fast become a bald, white, quivering, witless blob.

Too much copper in your mix and you go into free radical overload, damaging your DNA code and disrupting your body's ability to make the exact duplicates of the proteins necessary to maintain your skeleton, brain and organs. You become a bald, pink, putrescent, witless blob.[1,2]

Problem is, too much copper is only a little more than too little. And don't let ignorant medicine men fool you that anyone knows the right amount. In 1971, the World Health Organization declared that a daily copper intake of 0.5 mg per kilogram bodyweight should not cause toxic effects.[3] For an 80 kg (176 lb) person that's a whopping 40 mg of copper per day.

In 1977, the US National Research Council backed way off and cautioned that an *occasional* copper intake of 10 mg per day is probably safe for humans.[4] By 1989 the RDA Committee recommended a safe and adequate copper intake of 1.5 – 3.0 mg per day.[5] And Health Canada, who seem to want Canadians pale and docile, reduced their recommended copper to 1.0 – 2.0 mg per day.[6] You can see from these shenanigans that, over the last 30 years, estimates of safe copper intakes range from 2.0 – 40.0 mg, which doesn't do a lot to strengthen our faith in health politicians.

American men eat an average of about 1.2 mg of copper per day, American women 0.9 mg.[5] Metabolic balance studies, however, show that even sedentary men require 1.6 mg, per day for basic functions.[5] The 1995 RDI is 2.0 mg which seems to be about the true minimum requirement. By that standard most folk are in copper deficit. Don't be one of them.

Copper For Athletes

Because of its wide use in energy processes, hemoglobin formation, and antioxidant defenses, exercise raises copper

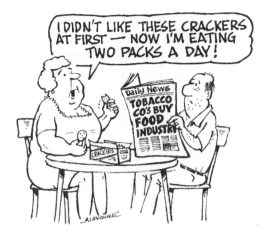

requirements substantially. Unfortunately, despite the claims of some researchers, we have no idea how much is optimal.[7] Estimates in athletes are based on **serum copper levels**, which do not reflect tissue levels or copper use[1,2] or levels of the copper-containing enzyme **ceruloplasmin.** Ceruloplasmin levels do decline with intense exercise[8], but this enzyme is also radically changed by hormonal disruption and inflammation that occur during exercise, so the copper may be going to other tissues.[9] Also, most studies to date are short-term measures before and after exercise, so findings are suspect as a measure of copper status.

In one of the a rare long-term studies, expert on copper, Henry Lucaski, at the US Department of Agriculture, found no overall change in ceruloplasmin copper of female swimmers over a whole competitive season.[10] But he had no way of telling whether their copper was in deficit to begin with, and they may have been simply operating at a sub-optimal level of function. Nor did he have any accurate measure of the daily amount of copper they were eating or absorbing.

The problem of determining copper intake and absorption illustrates a general principle which applies to all minerals. Getting down to the nitty-gritty, calculations of intake and absorption of nutrients from reported food intake are wildly inaccurate. Copper for example, varies widely in samples of the same food, depending on the copper content of the soil it was grown in, the rainfall during the growing season, at what stage the food was harvested and numerous other factors. Only God knows how much copper that particular oyster or bean or potato on your plate contains.

To say that two ounces of roasted sunflower seeds contain 1 mg of copper, or a medium boiled potato 0.6 mg, can be more than 50% wrong. Yet, computer generated lists of such values are accepted as gospel tracts. These lists might tell you that an athlete's reported food contains, 1.727 mg per day of copper, as if dividing out the decimal places somehow lends accuracy. It's a crock that should not fool even research nerds lost in the gloom of uninspired research. Don't let it fool you.

Then there's the problem of mineral absorption capacity of the gut. Taking copper again as the example, the amount absorbed varies inversely with the amount eaten. Given ideal gut conditions, an athlete eating 1 mg of copper will absorb only about 50% of it. An athlete eating 10 mg of copper per day, however, will absorb only about 10%.[11]

Throw some of the popular high-fructose corn syrup into the food and copper absorption drops even lower. Zinc also whacks copper absorption. And if you add high vitamin C, copper absorption declines to a minimum.[12] So well-fed athletes, who eat moderate fructose, high zinc and high vitamin C diets, need a lot more copper to get their ration.

Where does all this leave you? Hopefully convinced that we have done our homework. Based on all the above plusses and minuses, the Colgan Institute uses daily supplements of 1.0 – 5.0 mg of copper as **copper gluconate** with athletes. Most seem well supplied at the middle of this range. But hold the presses. We are still waiting to hear the fat lady sing about copper and many other minerals. Until then our supplemental range is a best guess. Toxicity – nil.

IODINE

Iodine forms part of your thyroid hormones **thyroxine** and **triodothyronine**.[1] Because your thyroid is a major controller of energy processes, you better get enough of it. Mild iodine deficiency causes hypothyroidism, and severe deficiency causes a complex of diseases that show themselves most obviously as an enlarged thyroid or goiter and mental retardation.

Seafood is an abundant source of iodine, providing as much as 4.5 mg per gram in some dried seaweeds used as Japanese foods. Used occasionally these seaweeds are fine, but make them a staple in your diet and you would quickly get thyrotoxicosis from excessive iodine.

The range between too little iodine and too much is wide. The RDA and 1995 RDI are both 150 mcg per day, which is sufficient to prevent deficiency in sedentary folk. With iodized salt and the iodine-containing chemicals used in large-scale bread making, the average intake in the US is above the RDI. Males get about 250 mcg of iodine per day and females 170 mcg.[3]

Iodine for Athletes

No one knows how much iodine athletes need. Sweat and urine are both potent sources of iodine loss from the body, and the rate of iodine loss is directly proportional to how much you sweat and how

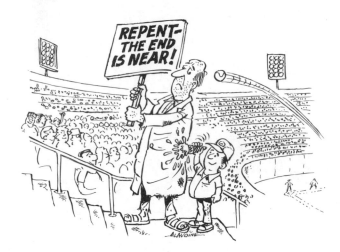

much you pee. Training in a temperate environment, you lose 40 mcg of iodine per liter or sweat, up to 150 mcg of iodine per day.[4,5] And, because athletes drink more than sedentary folk, urine losses of iodine are correspondingly greater.

Athletes who train in coastal regions and also eat a diet high in seafood have no worries. We have analyzed the iodine in their diets. It ranges from 440 – 1850 mcg per day. In inland areas of the US, in athletes who avoid seafood, iodine intake ranges from 180 - 496 mcg. Some of these folk need iodine supplementation. Recent research also indicates that iodine intake in some athletes is below the RDI.[6]

Iodine status is sometimes measured using **serum iodine**. It doesn't mean diddley, because iodine in the blood does not reflect tissue iodine status except in severe deficiency. A reasonable measure is **urinary excretion of iodine per gram of creatinine**. We like to see athletes above 60 mcg per gram.

It's easy to get iodine by eating iodized salt which provides 75 mcg per gram. But for athletes who wisely avoid excess salt, the Colgan Institute uses daily supplements of 150 – 300 mcg of iodine as **potassium iodide** in cases where the diet is not plentiful in iodine. Iodine is not toxic up to 2000 mcg per day.[7]

18

CHROMIUM

In 1955, Walter Mertz of the US Dept of Agriculture was the first to show that **trivalent chromium** is essential for insulin metabolism.[1] By the '70s, because of its potentiation of insulin, chromium was established as an essential element for carbohydrate, fat and protein metabolism, glucose control and muscle growth.[2,3]

Despite these and other well-defined functions, the shiny metal never made the RDA list, because no one had any idea how much was necessary for human health. In 1989, the RDA committee tentatively recommended an "estimated safe and adequate daily dietary intake" (ESADDI) of 50 – 200 mcg of chromium per day.[2] Sounds OK except that nutrition researchers all know that ESADDI more accurabtely signifies, "estimating safe amounts directly by divine inspiration." By 1995, the RDI was reduced to 120 mcg per day.

The numbers are academic anyway because hardly anyone gets that much. American chromium intake is only 33 mcg per day for men and 25 mcg for women.[4] And two ideal diets designed by dieticians to be complete in every essential nutrient contained only 62 mcg and 89 mcg of chromium per day.[5] If health professionals, with their research grants on the line, can't select a diet with sufficient chromium, then what chance have you or I with our variable day-to-day food.

Chromium is widely dispersed in foods but also widely variable, even in the same food. Sugar cane for example, contains plentiful chromium. The romantic might like to think it was designed in by Nature to help metabolize the sugar when it is eaten. But white table sugar has 90% of its chromium removed. Commercial greed is devoid of romance. Whole grains are also good sources of chromium, but processed white flours contain very little.[6] In out ever increasingly processed diet, most of the chromium is long gone.

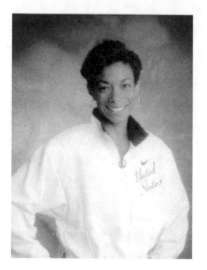

1500, 3000 and 5000 meter champion and many time Olympian, Regina Jacobs has used the best of nutrition with a Colgan Program to continue to extend her long career into her late 30s.

Diabetes Rampant

If most folk today are short of chromium, wouldn't they show it by developing insulin resistance and eventually diabetes? Yes they would — and it's happening in spades. In 1988 the World Health Organisation reported that low chromium intakes throughout the world are linked with incidence of diabetes, and warned us all that, without decisive action, incidence would skyrocket.[7]

As usual, different countries disagreed as to their share of responsibility, and, more pertinent, their share of the cost for providing sufficient chromium, so nothing has been done. By 1995 the worldwide incidence of diabetes had escalated to **135 million**, almost all of it adult-onset diabetes, and therefore largely preventable. By 2025 the projected number of diabetics is **300 million.**[8]

Chromium deficiency is not the only cause, but it's a big piece of the pie. More than half of all patients with glucose intolerance and incipient adult-onset diabetes become well again with simple chromium supplementation. Even apparently normal subjects improve their insulin metabolism.[2,9] And, with the most bioavailable form of chromium, **chromium picolinate**, Raymond Press at Mercy Hospital in San Diego has shown that some long-time insulin-dependent diabetics can reduce their need for insulin.[10]

Chromium For Athletes

Once chromium is mobilized for use by the body it cannot be saved from urine, because human kidneys do not have the mechanism to reabsorb it.[11] Richard Anderson and colleagues have shown repeatedly that exercise uses a ton of chromium. In one representative study, urinary loss of chromium increased five-fold after a six-mile run.[12] And the harder you train the more you lose.[13] Overall daily loss of chromium in athletes is about double that of sedentary folk.[14]

Convinced by this and similar research, researchers have warned that athletes may be short of chromium.[15] Some nig-nogs acknowledge the shortage, but still advise athletes get their chromium from a good diet, even though they are well aware that they could not themselves select a practical diet that contains sufficient chromium.[16]

There is yet no reliable way to assess chromium status and no human norms. We know from several studies, and our own cases, that animals and athletes supplemented with 200 - 800 mcg per day of chromium picolinate develop a little more muscle and a little less bodyfat.[17,18] Both effects are indicative of more efficient insulin metabolism. I especially like the studies that use chromium picolinate to grow leaner pigs. The porkers don't even know they are in a study, so they can't cheat.[19]

There are oodles of different chromium supplements offered in the marketplace. All those labeled "GTF" for "glucose tolerance factor" are bogus. Walter Mertz proposed the existence of a chemical complex he called GTF in 1955, but it has never been identified.

There are also some products that use the word "chromate" in literature and advertising. Chromate is a toxic hexavalent form of chromium firmly linked with bronchial cancer.[2] Despite use of the name, no supplement products are permitted to contain this poison.

The best form of chromium is chromium picolinate. It is five-fold better absorbed than the common supplement form chromium chloride, and is the only form shown to have beneficial effects in overt diabetes.

Studies by Leigh Broadbent and colleagues at the US Department of Agriculture, show that chromium picolinate is also better absorbed and retained in the human body than the other popular supplement form chromium polynicotinate. And recent research by Richard Anderson has refuted malicious claims of toxicity by commercial rivals, giving chromium picolinate a clean bill of health.[21] It is the only form we use with individual athletes.

The Colgan Institute uses daily supplements of 200 - 800 mcg of chromium as chromium picolinate with athletes. Most appear well supplied with 200 – 400 mcg. We have found no toxicity with this range in 16 years of use.

19

SELENIUM

Glutathione is one of your main endogenous antioxidants. Combined with **selenium**, it forms two antioxidant enzymes called **glutathione peroxidases**. These enzymes neutralize the highly toxic free radical, hydrogen peroxide (H_2O_2), a free radical that is increased manyfold by exercise, into harmless water (H_2O). The enzymes cannot function properly unless you eat sufficient selenium.[1,2]

Studies on humans are practically non-existent. But in animals, intense exercise causes large increases in glutathione peroxidase activity,[3,4] indicating that increased use of selenium can combat free radicals. And animals that are made selenium deficient and forced to exercise, show indicators of severe muscle damage by free radicals.[5]

Research in Keshan Province in China in 1979, showed that a prevalent form of heart disease there, called Keshan disease, was mainly caused by a diet chronically deficient in selenium, because of the low selenium levels in the soils.[6] This disease also occurs in other areas low in selenium, including New Zealand, parts of Australia and certain areas of the US. In 1981 I reported the low levels of selenium in 10 states plus the District of Columbia.[7] In many cases simple selenium supplementation *cures* Keshan disease.

Reacting to this evidence, and the amount of selenium required to prevent Keshan disease, the RDA Committee finally admitted selenium to the list in 1989, with an RDA of 70 mcg for men and 55 mcg for women.[8] These amounts are currently well provided by the average American diet.

In New Zealand, however, average selenium intake is only 29 mcg per day, insufficient to prevent disease.[9] It is a continuing but silent indictment of New Zealand health authorities, that human access to selenium supplements is still restricted there, while the sheep that country is so famous for, have selenium carefully added to their fodder.

Recent studies have shown that exposure to the **coxsackievirus** is also a causative factor in Keshan disease,[10] prompting researchers to look for other measures of selenium nutrition. Current flavor of the month is **glutathione peroxidase saturation**, that is the dose of selenium at which the level of these enzymes plateaus.[11]

Glutathione peroxidase saturation is a very oversimplified criterion for four reasons. First, numerous nutrients in addition to selenium participate in the manufacture of glutathione and its enzymes in your body.[12] So they may plateau for many reasons. Second, these enzyme levels are only affected by severe selenium deficiency.[13] Third, new selenium functions in the human body are being discovered literally every year, including involvement in genetic decoding and thyroid function.[14,15] Fourth, new research shows that selenium is also strongly involved in prevention of certain types of cancer. No one has any idea of the ideal amount of selenium to meet these needs.[16,17]

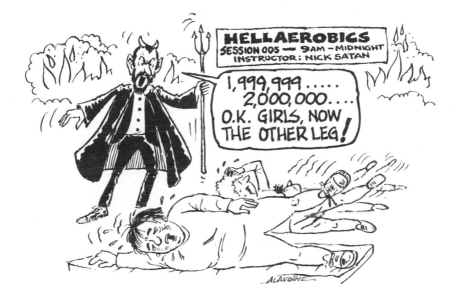

Selenium For Athletes

Well-fed rats forced to exercise show increased levels of glutathione peroxidase and other measures that indicate mobilization of antioxidant defenses.[4,5] But if you make the rats selenium deficient beforehand, glutathione peroxidase levels decline with exercise indicating a failure of antioxidant defenses.[18] So it is likely that additional selenium is required to combat the uncontrolled oxidation caused by exercise.

The little evidence we have on athletes shows no effects, primarily because they were not made selenium deficient beforehand and the exercise used was not sufficiently long or intense.[19] In any case, as noted above, you have to be mighty short of selenium for exercise to whack glutathione peroxidase sufficiently to reach significance in an experiment. So all we know for sure is that intense exercise mobilizes glutathione defenses.

After considering all the research to date, especially the need to prevent disease, we use supplements of **l-selenomethionine** with athletes. We use this organic form of selenium bound to the amino acid methionine because, in appropriate amounts, it is non-toxic. The inorganic form, sodium selenite that is commonly used in commercial supplements, is very toxic. Long-term use of even 1.0 mg per day of sodium selenite has caused selenium poisoning in rare cases.[8] Don't eat it.

The Colgan Institute uses daily supplements of 100 – 600 mcg of selenium as **l-selenomethionine** with athletes. Most appear well supplied towards the lower end of this range. We have found zero toxicity with this range of l-selenomethionine in 18 years of use.

20

MANGANESE & MOLYBDENUM

All animals including humans require manganese for proper formation of bone and cartilage and for insulin and glucose metabolism. It also forms an important part of **manganese superoxide dismutase**, the main antioxidant enzyme that guards the mitochondria of your cells.[1] These little structures, shaped like slater bugs, were once parasitic bacteria in the cells. They evolved into symbiotes and eventually became part of the human genome. They are the critters that perform the miraculous transfer of the energy from the sun that has been stored in food, to your flesh. Manganese is essential to protect the mitochondria from damage by the free radicals that the process of energy transfer creates.

Manganese occurs in most plant foods especially black tea and whole grains. The average manganese intake in America is about 2.7 mg per day for men and 2.2 mg for women.[2] These levels of intake yield a fairly constant level of manganese in human tissues, which some researchers take to mean that US manganese nutrition is adequate.[3]

Attempts to define manganese requirements using balance studies, that is, manganese in/manganese out, have all failed.[3] These short-term studies tell us only that it takes about the average intake to maintain a certain range of manganese in the body. They say nothing about adequate levels for optimal glucose metabolism, bone growth or superoxide dismutase function.[4] Acting again on divine inspiration, in 1989 the RDA Committee recommended an ESADDI for manganese of 2.0 – 5.0 mg per day. The 1995 RDI reduced the amount to 2.0 mg per day.

Manganese For Athletes

Because of their larger turnover of bone and cartilage, their greater metabolism of glucose and their greater demand on antioxidant defense systems, athletes likely need more manganese than sedentary souls. But no one knows how much more. Recent studies on the diets of elite Soviet athletes in intense training, showed that more manganese was being excreted than occurred in their food. Supplementation with manganese restored the balance.[5]

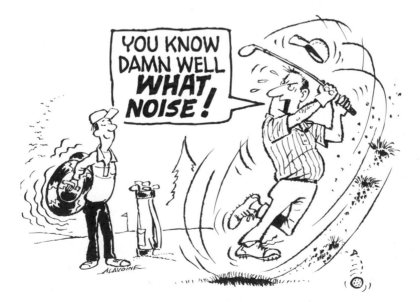

Manganese is a benign element judging from animal studies. The toxic oral dose for humans is likely over 10 mg per day.[1,6] No toxicity was found in subjects who habitually consumed 8 – 9 mg per day.[3] Your body is also reasonable protected against manganese poisoning by its low absorption rate and rapid elimination in bile.[7] The Colgan Institute uses supplements of 2.0 – 5.0 mg of manganese as **manganese gluconate** with athletes. Most appear well supplied at the lower end of this range. Toxicity of range – nil.

Molybdenum

You need molybdenum for a number of essential enzymes, including **aldehyde oxidase, sulfite oxidase** and **xanthine oxidase**[1] involved in sulfur metabolism, amino acid metabolism and uric acid production. Without sufficient molybdenum you grow poorly and die early.[1,2] Yet some learned texts on sports nutrition hardly mention this essential element.[3]

Molybdenum varies widely in foods depending on the molybdenum content of the soil on which they were grown[4] And we know virtually nothing about its bioavailability from different foods, except that it varies widely.[5] So estimates of average intakes of Americans, calculated from reported diets, are all suspect as measures of molybdenum status. The best estimate to date is that of Pennington and colleagues from the FDA Total Diet Study. They reported average molybdenum intake at 109 mcg per day for males and 76 mcg for females. Based on these figures the RDA Committee "provisionally recommended" 75 – 250 mcg per day.[6] The 1995 RDI reduced this to 75 mcg.

Molybdenum For Athletes

No tests yet exist for molybdenum status. Young men fed doses from 22 – 1496 mcg per day of supplemental molybdenum showed progressively greater excretion of molybdenum in urine and feces, suggesting that the body has a protective mechanism against molybdenum excess. All doses were also very efficiently absorbed (90%)

and equally efficiently excreted without adverse effects.[7] A small amount of data on molybdenum deficiency in humans, suggests that the RDI of 75 mcg may be insufficient. In these subjects it took 160 mcg per day of supplemental molybdenum to reverse the symptoms.[6]

Frank molybdenum toxicity occurs at intakes of about 10 mg per day, raising uric acid levels and causing gout-like disease. Even 1.0 mg per day may interfere with copper metabolism.[6] So don't eat a lot of it.

New functions of molybdenum are being reported almost annually, so the jury is still out on how much you need.[8] We have no data at all on the needs of athletes. Because of the new functions, however, and because optimal amino acid metabolism is crucial for growth of muscle and strength, the Colgan Institute uses daily supplements of 100 – 300 mcg of molybdenum as **ammonium molybdate** with athletes. Toxicity of this range – nil.

SILICON & BORON

The element **silicon** (popularly called silica) has a bad, though largely underserved, reputation when used in breast implants. But, in the right amounts, it is an essential element for normal growth of human bone and cartilage, nails and hair.[1,2]

Foods highest in silicon are whole oats, barley and rice and the herb horsetail. No one knows how much silicon is optimum, but dietary intakes in America vary from 20 – 50 mg per day. With an approximate 10% bioavailability, the amount of silicon absorbed is about 1 – 5 mg.[3] Average daily intake in America is about 40 mg for men and 19 mg for women.[4]

Silicon For Athletes

Whether these average daily intakes meet the needs of athletes is unknown. But studies of male Russian elite athletes indicate that silicon excretion increases big-time with heavy exercise. These researchers recommend supplementation of highly trained athletes with 30 - 35 mg of silicon per day.[5]

There are no tests of silicon status worth a damn. Because of its involvement in bone and cartilage growth, the Colgan Institute uses supplements of 10 – 30 mg of silicon, as an extract from the herb **Equisetum arvense**, with athletes. Most seem well supplied around the middle of this range. Toxicity – nil.

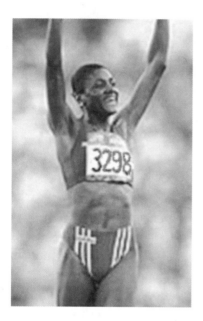

Marie Perec shows how well correct nutrition and training benefit the human body.

Boron

Boron was first shown to be an essential nutrient for normal growth in chickens in 1981.[1] Since then numerous studies have found that boron is probably essential for normal production of steroid hormones in humans, especially hormones involved in muscle growth and in calcium, phosphorus and magnesium metabolism for bone growth and maintenance.[2]

Boron is found in numerous foods but most plentifully in peanuts, nuts, wine, raisins and dates. In 1987 the Colgan Institute did an analysis of a good, mixed diet. Mean boron intake was 1.9 mg per day.[3] A more comprehensive analysis of average American diets in 1999 reported male intakes of 0.4 – 2.4 mg per day, with an average of 1.02 mg, and female intakes of 0.3 – 1.9 mg per day, with an average of 0.86 mg.[4]

No one knows how much boron you need. New functions are being discovered regularly, including optimization of estrogen and testosterone levels and regulation of essential pathways using a variety of **nucleotides** and **serine protease** enzymes.[5,6]

Boron For Athletes

Expert in trace mineral nutrition, Forrest Neilsen at the US Department of Agriculture, Nutrition Research Center in Grand Forks North Dakota, recently reviewed the evidence that excess boron is promptly excreted, and that adult intakes of boron are safe up to 13 mg per day. The research called for establishment of a dietary reference range, with concerns that the current average intake of less than 1.0 mg may be inadequate. Studies have reported boron deficiency in humans and a variety of animals.[7]

Women show improved calcium metabolism when supplemented with 3 mg of boron per day.[8] Supplements of 10 mg per day cause a large increase in plasma estrogen, even though about 80% of the dose is promptly passed into urine.[9] In one of the few studies with female athletes, boron supplementation for one year increased bone mineral density.[10]

Despite the hype in muscle magazines, boron supplements do not increase testosterone levels in healthy males. Testosterone production is under multiple tight controls. Though boron is involved, it would raise testosterone levels only in the case of boron deficiency.[11]

After reviewing all research to date, the Colgan Institute uses supplements of 3.0 – 6.0 mg of boron as **boron citrate** and **aspartate** with athletes. Toxicity of range – nil.

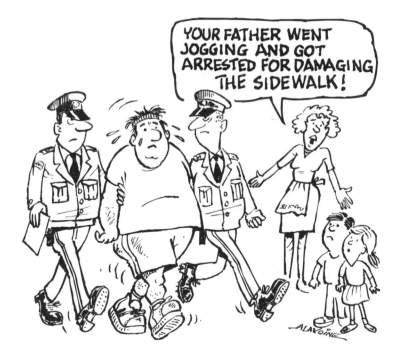

22

VANADIUM & ARSENIC

Because of its hardness and resistance to corrosion, the grey metal vanadium is commonly mixed with iron and other minerals to form tough steel alloys used in machines and tools. It also appears to be an essential part of the mineral mix that forms a tough human body. Since 1973 a ton of evidence has shown that microgram amounts of vanadium are essential for normal health and growth in a variety of mammals.[1]

In 1985, vanadium hit the spotlight. A report in the prestigious journal *Science*, showed that if you put large doses of supplemental vanadium in the drinking water of rats that have been made diabetic, their blood sugar returned to normal.[2] Diabetes researchers seized upon oral vanadium as a possible simple alternative to injected insulin.

Confirming experiments quickly followed[3], but the amounts of vanadium required to normalize blood sugar proved toxic and killed many of the animals involved.[4,5] More recent studies using smaller doses have shown less toxicity.[6] Meanwhile the supplement industry, sensed the big bucks that could be made for any product that reduced blood sugar and stabilized insulin, and thus might enhance muscle growth and fat loss. They rushed to market with pills containing up to 100 mg vanadyl sulfate led by wild claims of anabolic effects.

Fortunately absorption of vanadyl sulfate through the gut is very low, so few cases of human poisoning resulted. Despite loud claims of muscle-pumping success by strutting, steroid bozos, well paid for their sideshow, vanadyl sulfate slipped quietly into oblivion. It still exists in the marketplace only because the ignorant will always part with folding green for anything that even hints of a shortcut to muscle power.

The evidence that really damns vanadyl sulfate is that diabetics don't use it. And there's no evidence over the last 16 years that even one human diabetic has been helped by it. Some of the original researchers have now turned to less toxic and better absorbed forms of vanadium. One of these, **bismaltolato-oxovanadium** may have a future as an adjunctive drug in treatment of diabetes.[3] But it has nothing to do with vanadium as an essential mineral.

Vanadium For Athletes

Vanadium occurs in a wide range of foods. The average American diet contains 10 – 60 micrograms per day.[7] In these amounts it appears to activate some enzymes involved with insulin receptors called **serine and threonine kinases**. So there is a connection with insulin and its functions.[2]

No one knows how much vanadium is optimal, but it is likely to be less than 500 micrograms. There are no studies on the vanadium needs of athletes. The Colgan Institute uses daily supplements of 25 – 100 mcg of vanadium as vanadyl sulfate with athletes. Toxicity of range – nil.

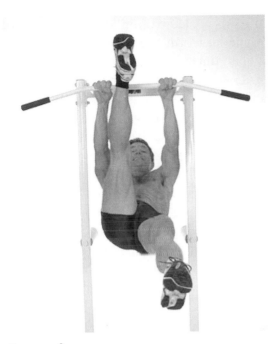

Michael Colgan demonstrating the hanging vertical scissors abdominal exercise from the Colgan Power Program.

Arsenic

Folk at my lectures seem surprised when I list arsenic as an essential mineral. It conjures up Agatha Christie images of sinister old ladies lacing tea with arsenic to poison unwary guests. Yet you eat minute amounts of this element every day, and your body wouldn't work properly without it. Remember it's always the dose that makes any chemical either a benefit or a poison. Studies show that diets without arsenic retard growth in chickens, rats, goats and pigs.[1] No human studies yet, but some brave soul will do one before long.

Seafood and rice contain the highest levels of arsenic[2,3] but the latest FDA Total Diet Study found appreciable levels in a quarter of all foods tested.[2] It was not in there as a pollutant introduced by man, but as a natural part of the food. The average adult intake of arsenic in America is about 50 micrograms per day.[2]

The story of arsenic provides a great illustration of the way in which naturally occurring chemicals became essential to the human body. It's likely that ancient foods contained similar natural levels of arsenic as foods do today, when our worm-like ancestors wriggled in the primaeval swamps. At that time we were little more than a segmented tube with a bulge at one end. This tube spent practically all its time finding and consuming sufficient edibles to keep it alive, a task that quickly wore it out. Fortunately, whenever it was full of food, it could take time off from the hunt to beget baby tubes to keep the whole process going. All the while arsenic was along for the ride.

Over countless millennia the bulge end developed into a head, with unbelievably complex mechanisms called eyes and ears, and the tube end grew arms and legs. And it incorporated the strong stimulatory properties of arsenic to help it grow. Now it could snaffle its food much more easily, in just a fraction of each day. Just lying around like a slug the rest of the time was very boring. So it invented other activities.

The best invention was blowing air out its intake hole to make weird noises at other tubes nearby, mostly to tell them, "I'm a nicer, stronger, prettier tube than you." But sound doesn't carry very far and quickly fades. So, after a while the tube invented another great activity. It began to make marks on papyrus leaves and other materials. Now it could tell distant tubes and even future generations how superior it was. In a wink of the evolutionary eye, books encircled the globe.

Over all that time and development of the body, it's very likely that human tubes learned to use the unique properties of arsenic for beneficial functions. We are not quite smart enough yet to find out exactly what those functions are. Until we do, the Colgan Institute does not use arsenic with athletes, (except for certain individuals for whom we have developed an intense dislike).

23

FLUORIDE

In 1942, a study reported that children who lived in areas of the US with low levels of **fluoride** in the water had a lot of dental caries.[1] That was the start of the fluoride wars. After confirming studies, the US Dental Association recommended fluoridation of water supplies in areas of low natural fluoride.[2]

Rightly fearful of big government putting drugs in the water for whatever reason, millions of people objected. Nevertheless, fluoridation went ahead, and the objections only served to fuel overstatement of the benefits of fluoride. Numerous local authorities then dumped too much fluoride into their water, or put it in water that already contained enough fluoride. This fluoride overdose caused **fluorosis** in thousands of children, fluoride toxicity which gave them permanently mottled teeth. What the dentists in these areas lost on the swings of declining dental fillings, they more than gained on the roundabouts of porcelain caps to cover up the mess.

Fluoride provides a good example of a general principle of nutrition. As with all minerals it's the dose that makes it a nutrient or a poison. In a previous book I called fluoride by its correct elemental name **fluorine**. The president of a big bookstore chain in Britain refused the book because he had looked up fluorine in a dictionary and it said "a poisonous green gas." It is, but in small amounts of its ionized form **fluoride**, it is also an essential element for the formation of bone and tooth enamel.[2,3]

Too much fluoride, however, damages bones and teeth, kidneys, and nerve function.[3] And the gap between sufficient or too much, nutrient or poison, is pretty small. Some children show evidence of fluorosis at doses of only 2 mg of fluoride per day.[4] Yet some uninformed dentists still recommend fluoride pills that raise total fluoride intake way beyond this level.

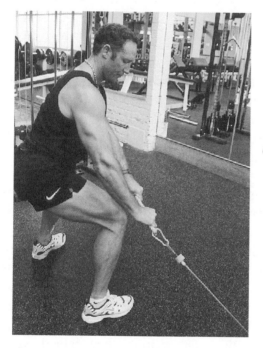

Top trainer
Lee Parore
demonstrates core
agility and
coordination
exercises on the
Colgan Power
Program.

Fluoride For Athletes

Fluoride occurs widely in food and water. The range of intake from average US diets is 0.9 – 1.7 mg per day, the lower figure usually in low fluoride areas. A recent food analysis in Canada estimated fluoride intake at 1.76 mg per day.[5] From the data on dental caries, the RDA Committee set the adult ESADDI (estimating safe amounts by divine inspiration) for fluoride at 1.5 – 4.0 mg per day with a maximum level for children of 2.5 mg per day.

Individual fluoride intake is a bit more complicated. If you use teflon-coated pots and pans for example, you also get an inadvertent supplement of fluoride, because teflon contains high amounts and releases it readily. If you use aluminum pots and pans, you lose fluoride, because aluminum grabs it out of the food and cooking water.[6]

Habitual diet is also important. If you habitually drink black tea like the English, this potent source of fluoride can provide over 1 mg per day. Coffee drinkers, however, get negligible fluoride from their favorite brew.[7]

No test exists for fluoride status and no one knows how much is optimum. The best indicator we have is healthy white teeth. Fluoride is taken into tooth enamel lifelong.[2] Don't believe uninformed health professionals who tell you that, once formed, tooth enamel doesn't change. Everything in your body changes all the time. That's why what you eat is so important to maintain and grow your structure.

Until we learn a lot more about fluoride the Colgan Institute doesn't use it with athletes, and doesn't use fluoridated water either. It seems to be the right decision. Numerous athletes who have been on our nutrition programs for a decade or more have exceptional dental health. And, except for a tooth broken in an accident, I haven't had a filling in 27 years.

"Today's teaching is lost in an ocean of words. Real knowledge is always experiential. You have to do. There is no way I can tell you the taste of honey. You have to experience it upon your tongue."

- Michael Colgan
Program Your Mind Lecture Series, 2001

COBALT, TIN, NICKEL, GERMANIUM

Some plant foods contain tiny amounts of **cobalt**-containing chemicals that can be converted into vitamin B_{12} by bacterial synthesis in your gut. But it's a difficult process, which is why ruminant animals such as cows and *strict* vegetarians are often short of vitamin B_{12}[1]. The rest of us get our vitamin B_{12} mostly preformed along with its cobalt, from meats and dairy foods and vitamin supplements. Cobalt has no other known function except as part of vitamin B_{12}, so there is no need for this element by itself.[1]

Cobalt is useful pharmacologically in treatment of cyanide poisoning, as it binds readily with cyanide.[2] Most folk are unaware that, for stability purposes, the commercial form of vitamin B_{12}, **cyanocobalamin**, is a complex of cyanide and cobalamin. The cyanide is removed and discarded in your gut and the remainder converted to active vitamin B_{12}. People who take multi-milligram supplements of vitamins B_{12} are under the mistaken belief that it boosts their energy, get more than a little cyanide along with their placebo. The cyanide might account for the high they report from their B_{12} overdoses. Use of cobalt with athletes as part of the vitamin B_{12} is covered under vitamins ahead.

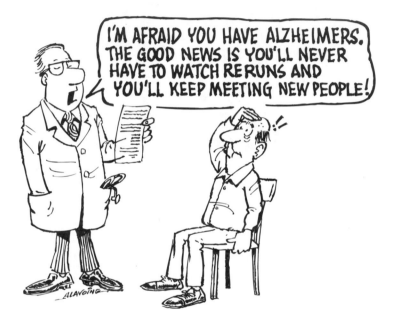

Tin

Tin is a bit of a mystery metal. Forrest Nielsen at the US Dept of Agriculture has shown that animals fed a tin-free diet grow poorly.[3] So it seems to have some function as a nutrient. But rats fed larger than normal doses of tin, show loss of iron and disruption of zinc and copper metabolism.[4,5] Medical studies show many toxic effects of tin, including disruption of copper, zinc and iron metabolism, reduction of glutathione levels and interference with multiple enzyme functions.[6]

On an unprocessed food diet, tin intake is usually less than 1 mg per day. But processed food in tinfoil or tinned packs, such as pizza, and canned foods, may leach enough tin to give you a toxic dose of 10 mg per day.[6] Avoiding the tin is yet another good reason for ditching processed glop from your diet.

It will be a long time before science figures out whether tin is a necessary element for humans. Meanwhile, we would like to add a new designation for it and other questionable trace elements to the RDA, DRI, EAR and other tomfoolery put out as nutrition standards by the US Academy of Sciences. Ours is "tolerable daily intake" or TDI. For tin the TDI seems to be about one milligram.

Nickel

Another silver mystery metal, nickel is nice to look at and widely used in metals in contact with food. Forrest Nielsen has also shown retarded growth in numerous species of animals fed a **nickel**-free diet.[3] But no one has found a function for nickel in the human system except toxicity. The natural level of nickel in foods is about 230 mcg per day in Canadian diets[7] and the same in French diets.[8] So all we have to go on is that level as a presumed tolerable daily intake (TDI).

Germanium

I am including **germanium** here because, for a few years, some dopey Japanese studies were commercially hyped to suggest that this element had essential healthful functions in humans. Hopefully, I and other scientists poured enough scorn on that notion to make it vanish like the smoke it was. But germanium supplements are still around to fool the uninformed.

All science knows about germanium in human nutrition, is that it readily causes kidney damage and persists in the human system for long periods after supplementation is stopped.[9] The presumed tolerable daily intake (TDI) is about 1.5 mg per day, the level at which germanium occurs naturally in average diets. Avoid it if you can. Take germanium supplements only if you have a strong desire to be chronically ill.

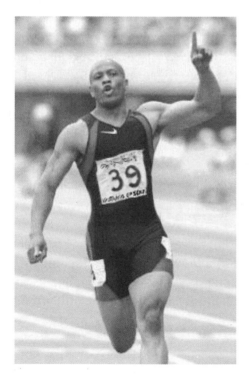

*Maurice Green flying.
The fastest man on the
planet.*

25

VITAMINS
IN ACTION

Even college textbooks used to state that athletes need no greater amounts of vitamins than sedentary folk, and are well covered by the RDA, which they should get from a good diet. As you will see ahead, a ton of new evidence has buried that hokum forever.[1] We know now that all sorts of physical stresses increase vitamin requirements. Even the ultra-conservative RDA for vitamin C, has been increased by 67% for anyone subject to the stress of tobacco smoke or similar air pollution.[1] Athletes put their bodies under far heavier stress than smokers.

We also used to see similar hokum that athletes eat more than sedentary folk, so would naturally get any greater amount of vitamins they might need from the increased food intake. No way! As I have documented in previous books, vitamins are very unevenly distributed in foods, and vary widely even in different samples of the same food.[2-4]

Vitamin content of foods is also decimated by modern food processing.[5] Oranges for example, that are picked green, then ripened by ethylene gas, and kept for weeks in storage, may have virtually no vitamin C left in them.[5] In 1998 the US National Academy of Sciences admitted that American food does not contain sufficient vitamins to supply even the RDA, and recommended that most folk should take vitamin supplements.[6]

Leaping upon this bandwagon, supplement carpetbaggers are touting all sorts of weird concoctions of vitamins and other substances as ergogenic, that is, providing a rapid, drug-like boost to sports performance. In a properly nourished body these witches' brews have never worked and never will. You **can** produce drug effects with mega-doses of vitamins. But they are very poor at the job, because your body recognizes them as building and maintenance materials, uses them accordingly, and eventually discards the excess. Meanwhile you upset the balance of your whole biochemical mix.

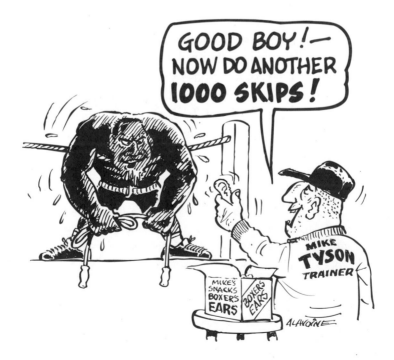

The Business of Vitamins

Vitamins work to give you an edge by combining with the effects of training to build better structure and function. That takes a long time. As a vital part of your plan to excel, you take your individual vitamin formula every single day, 365 days a year, year in, year out. Together with other nutrients, plus the right year-round training, the correct amounts of vitamins will gradually improve every cell of your body, until it performs like a god.

The real questions are: what constitutes the right amount of each vitamin for this task, and where do you get them? To answer these questions I will review the recent evidence on each vitamin under the following criteria:

- Major functions
- Food sources
- Are athletes deficient?
- How to measure status
- How much do athletes need?
- Toxicity

Let's get rolling, we have a lot of ground to cover.

*"Excellence never occurs
by accident."*

- Michael Colgan
Sports Lecture Series, 2000

26

VITAMIN A

Fat soluble vitamin A is essential for vision, growth, reproduction, skin, mucous membranes and immune function.[1] It provides the photosensitive pigments of the retina, which react to light somewhat like the film in an instant camera, enabling you to see moving pictures in your mind. The first symptom of vitamin A deficiency is impaired night vision. And it's a lot more common than many folk think.

Best food sources are the preformed vitamin A, **retinol,** in liver, fish liver oils and egg yolks, Next best is the potential vitamin A in **alpha-** and **beta-carotene**, and one or two others of the 500 or so different carotenoids that form the bright yellow to red pigments of fruits and vegetables. Most carotenoids have no potential vitamin A activity, but are important nutrients for other reasons. Tomatoes for example, are colored by the red carotenoid **lycopene**, which is a vital antioxidant in the body, but has no vitamin A activity.

We used to think that beta-carotene was easily absorbed and readily converted to retinol as the body required it. Recent research, however, suggests that only about 20% of beta-carotene may be absorbed and only a small fraction of that is converted to retinol.[2] Beta-carotene has other vital functions, however, some of which we cover in the chapters ahead on antioxidants and polyphenols.

Though the obsolete measure, international units (IU), still appears on food and supplement labels, vitamin A activity has been measured as **retinol equivalents** (RE) in science for at least 20 years. To make it easy:

> 1 RE = 10 IU from beta-carotene
> = 6 micrograms beta-carotene
> = 3.33 IU from retinol
> = 1 microgram retinol

The RDA and the 1995 RDI are both 1000 RE (3,333 IU) (male) and 800 RE (2,667 IU) (female). Because of the new evidence of poor absorption and conversion of carotenoids to vitamin A, vegetarians may require 30,000 IU of beta-carotene every day, just to meet the RDA for vitamin A.

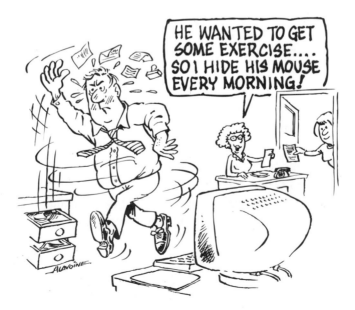

Vitamin A For Athletes

Research on athletes shows that strenuous exercise causes substantial release of vitamin A from the liver into the bloodstream, raising blood levels by 10 – 40%.[3] But because athletes are somewhat resistant to having their livers removed for analysis, there is no way to determine whether liver stores become seriously depleted. But studies of animals, whose rightful ownership of their bodyparts is seldom recognized in science, show that repeated bouts of daily strenuous exercise rapidly depletes liver vitamin A.[4] Overall, these findings on both rats and men, suggest that exercise increases requirements for vitamin A substantially.

It's difficult to know whether athletes are deficient in vitamin A, because most studies are based on total intake of vitamin A and carotenoids together, and do not measure blood levels. But one study of German national teams showed a range of serum retinol from 49.5 to 93.1 micrograms/dl. The level of deficiency at which medical symptoms start to occur is 20 micrograms/dl. We like to see athletes above 40 micrograms/dl.[5] This level can be achieved and maintained during heavy training by vitamin A intake of 1000 – 3000 RE per day (3,333 – 10,000 IU).

Don't take more vitamin A than the top of our range. Overdose can be very toxic and builds up in the liver with repeated supplementation. Toxicity begins at about 5,000 RE (16,667 IU).[6]

"L'homme se decouvre quand il se mesure avec l'obstacle."

- St Exupery

27

VITAMIN B1 THIAMIN

Water-soluble, and therefore quickly in and out of the body within 24 hours, **thiamin** is a vital component of energy metabolism. Thiamin is also required for metabolism of the essential branched-chain amino acids **leucine, isoleucine** and **valine**, and for manufacture of the long chain fatty acids that form most of your brain and other highly active tissues, and for the firing of every nerve in your body.[1] So you better get enough of it every day.

Best sources of thiamin are raw, fresh whole grains, beans and peas. But food processing, cooking and baking of breads and cereals destroys most of the thiamin.[2] Despite the thiamin fortification of so-called "enriched" breads and cereals, deficient intakes of thiamin are common in athletes, even at the tiny adult RDI level of 1.5 mg/day.[3,4]

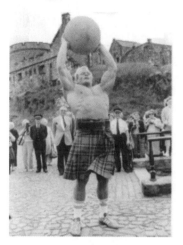

One of the world's strongest men that ever lived, Jon Paul Sigmarsson.

Thiamin For Athletes

You may need a lot more thiamin than the RDI. At the Colgan Institute, we have used the **erythrocyte transketolase thiamin pyrophosphate stimulation (TLPP)** assay to measure thiamin status for more than 20 years. An acceptable level for athletes is below 10% TLPP stimulation.[5] To maintain that level in many athletes requires a thiamin intake of only 10 mg/day. Because of genetic individuality, however, some odd bods require up to 150 mg/day to maintain thiamin status.

The Colgan Institute uses thiamin supplements with athletes of 10 – 150 mg/day. Thiamin is non-toxic to at least 500 mg/day.[6] Common vitamin supplements sold as "Stress B complexes may contain 50 – 100 mg. These amounts are higher than needed by most athletes, and there is no evidence whatsoever that they have any effect on "stress". But there is also no evidence they are harmful, High intakes of thiamin may even prove to be beneficial, because science continues to discover new facets of its multifaceted role in human performance.

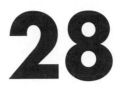

VITAMIN B2 RIBOFLAVIN

Water-soluble **riboflavin** is essential for the mitochondria of your cells to produce ATP from carbohydrates, fats and proteins, and in the formation of your vital endogenous antioxidant **glutathione**. The 1995 adult RDI for riboflavin is 1.7 mg. Athletes, however, use up to 20 times more energy than the sedentary folk for whom this standard was devised, and require more riboflavin both for the energy conversion process and to make glutathione to combat their increased levels of free radicals.[1]

Riboflavin is widely distributed in foods. Best sources are meats, fish, and dairy products. But riboflavin content of the same food can vary widely in different samples.[2] This variation may explain why some studies find well-fed athletes who are deficient in riboflavin, while others do not.[3,4]

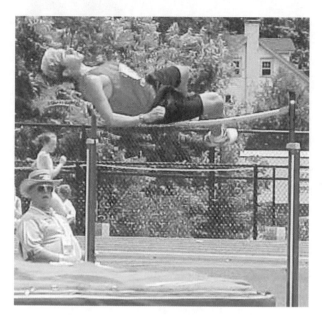

With correct nutrition, you too can fly like this young athlete at the USATF 2001 youth championships.

Riboflavin For Athletes

The best measure we have of riboflavin status reflects its essential functions in glutathione metabolism: the **erythrocyte glutathione reductase activity coefficient (EGRAC)**. We used to take an EGRAC of 1.25 or more as a sign of deficiency, but more recent evidence suggests that above 1.35 may be more accurate.[5] Reevaluating our measurements over the last two decades using the new criterion, indicates that some athletes we considered deficient were probably not.

The Colgan Institute uses supplements of riboflavin of 10 – 100 mg per day. Most athletes are probably well supplied at a supplementary intake of 10 mg per day. But we have measured some that need much greater amounts to achieve an acceptable EGRAC. Also, most of the research measurements of riboflavin status in athletes have been short-term and with only moderate exercise. In extreme stress conditions such as the intense training regimens of today, the biochemistry of the human body changes dramatically.

We know that riboflavin use increases with even very moderate exercise.[6] We know that it is essential for all energy production and for the body's antioxidant defense system. So it just doesn't sit right that intense exercise, which may use 20 times the energy of light exercise, and which has your antioxidant defense system working frantically to combat the greatly increased free radicals, requires only twice the riboflavin that satisfies Joe Slug slumping in front of the tube.

In the latest review, Manore of Arizona State University also documents other effects of exercise that may increase riboflavin needs: biochemical adaptations to training, increased levels of mitochondrial enzymes that require riboflavin, and increased riboflavin need for body maintenance and repair[7] So until there are some decent long-term studies that define riboflavin needs of athletes, we will continue to stick our necks out and recommend riboflavin to spare. Toxicity of our range —nil.[8]

"Never bolster your competitors' confidence by presenting a disorganised face to the world."

- Michael Colgan
Sports Lecture Series, 2002

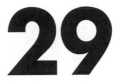

VITAMIN B3 NIACIN, NIACINAMIDE

Also known as nicotinic acid and nicotinamide, the two forms of vitamin B₃ are water-soluble and quickly excreted, so must be eaten every day for optimal health. Vitamin B₃ is not active in the human body until it is converted to two enzymes, **nicotinamide adenine dinucleotide (NAD)** and its phosphate **(NADP)**. These coenzymes are essential for the energy cycle, the manufacture of fats and proteins, and some 200 other enzymatic reactions.[1]

The human body can make some niacin from the essential amino acid tryptophan, but not sufficient for optimal health. In a typical synergistic action of the vitamins, conversion of tryptophan to niacin requires both riboflavin (vitamin B₂) and pyridoxine (vitamin B₆) to accomplish the task.[1]

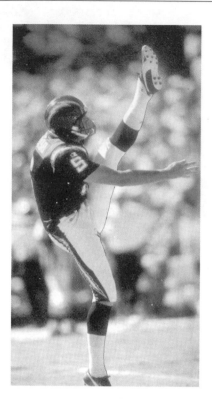

*Chargers kicker
Darren Bennett
shows the sort of
flexibility you
should aim for.*

The best food sources of preformed niacin are meats, fish, and poultry. Although whole grains contain substantial preformed niacin, most of it is not bioavailable.[1]

Niacin For Athletes

A lot of silly experiments have used mega-doses of niacin and niacinamide looking for so-called ergogenic effects on athletic performance. Overall they have reported enhanced use of glycogen but *reduced* performance.[2] Nevertheless, some athletes have been persuaded by distorted media reports of these studies to take excess niacin. All they get is a red, prickly face, both from embarrassment, and from the histamine release which causes a "niacin flush."

The biochemistry by which niacin reduces performance has been known since 1963. Muscle cannot store much fat and must get it for fuel from adipose cells. Both the release of fats from these cells, and use of the fats for fuel is under hormonal control. Excess niacin interferes with the hormonal cascade and inhibits use of fat.[3] So don't take too much of the stuff. One of those big, misnamed "anti-stress" B-complexes every day will both whack your performance and reduce your ability to lower bodyfat.

You can get a good idea of your niacin status with the urine test of **N-methylnicotinamide**. Expressed as mg/gram urine creatinine, a sufficient level is 3.0 or more. The 1995 RDI for niacin is 20 mg for adults. Athletes probably require more because of the heavy involvement of niacin in the energy cycle and in synthesis of fats and proteins. The Colgan Institute uses supplements of 25-50 mg niacin plus 20-100 niacinamide. Most athletes are well supplied at the lower end of these ranges. Toxicity of our ranges —nil.

"Life is not fair. Esteem is not given in proportion to worth, nor reward in proportion to effort. Put your faith in adventure and challenge. The key is timing."

- Michael Colgan
Sports Lecture Series, 2002

VITAMIN B6 PYRIDOXINE

Pyridoxine is a coenzyme for over 100 enzyme functions in humans. Most are essential to amino acid metabolism, therefore critical to optimum growth and repair of muscle. One pyridoxine-dependent enzyme especially important for athletes is **glycogen phosphorylase** which acts to break down muscle glycogen to fuel the energy cycle. The greater the glycogen use the greater the need for pyridoxine.

Because of its involvement in glycogen metabolism and in amino acid metabolism, pyridoxine requirements increase not only with energy use, but also with high protein diets, a necessary part of athletic nutrition. Even for sedentary folk on high protein diets, recent research shows that the 1995 RDI of 2.0 mg is far too low.[1]

Best food sources are wheat germ, fish, chicken and eggs. With such wide availability in foods used extensively by athletes, you might think deficiency unlikely. Research shows otherwise.

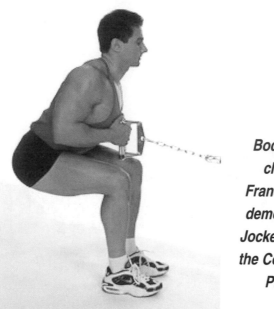

Bodybuilding champion Franco Cavaleri demonstrates a Jockey Row from the Colgan Power Program.

Pyridoxine For Athletes

Here are some representative examples. In two groups of runners measured at the Colgan Institute, 58% and 73% were pyridoxine deficient.[2] In 57 strength and speed/power athletes, 30% showed pyridoxine intake below the RDA, and 90% had whole blood levels of vitamin B_6 below the minimum reference level of 0.88 nmol/ml.[3] Most of a group of 16 female collegiate rowers were also found to have deficient pyridoxine intake, even when the reference value was set as only two-thirds of the RDA.[4] These and similar studies indicate that pyridoxine deficiency is common among athletes, even the well-fed.

Deficient pyridoxine intake is doubly bad because a pile of studies show that pyridoxine deficiency impairs performance, and that exercise uses pyridoxine like candy. A single marathon race, for example, uses at least 1.0 mg of pyridoxine.[3,7]

Unfortunately, we still don't have a good measure of pyridoxine status, and little idea of what amount might be optimal for athletes. The Colgan Institute uses **erythrocyte glutamic oxaloacetic transaminase (EGOT) activity in the presence and absence of pyridoxal-5-phosphate**. Athletes seem to be O.K. at an activity coefficient of 1.25 or less. But science still has a way to go to develop a definitive test.[6,9]

Deciding how much pyridoxine athletes need is made even more difficult by new evidence that this vitamin is intimately involved in stimulating the body's antioxidant defense system, especially the major endogenous antioxidant, glutathione.[8] As you will see in the chapter ahead, Antioxidant Armor, every athlete needs maximum protection against free radicals, and we are only just learning how to do it.[9]

For its wide range of functions crucial to athletes, the Colgan Institute uses 15 – 75 mg of pyridoxine per day. Most athletes are probably well supplied with 20 mg. Toxicity of our range — nil.

"Those who view life as a problem to be overcome, lack their own proper ballast. Seriousness is activity for the dullard. Clever people play."

- Henry Miller

31

VITAMIN B12 COBALAMIN

For stability purposes, the supplement form of vitamin B_{12} is almost always **cyanocobalamin**, which is converted in the body to three different forms, **hydroxycobalamin**, **adenosylcobalamin** and **methylcobalamin**. These babies are important for athletes in three main ways. First they are required for **erythropoiesis**, that is, formation of red blood cells, and hence for oxygen transport. Second, cobalamin functions to control the metabolic residue of use of fats as fuel. Third, even a minor deficiency of cobalamin inhibits the conversion of homocysteine back to methionine. (We cover the homocysteine cycle in the chapters ahead.)

The main sources of vitamin B_{12} are meats, eggs and milk. Vegetables and fruits don't contain B_{12}. Hence, vegetarians are often deficient. I mean *real* vegetarians, not the pseudo-ovo-lacto prickmedainties who sniff condescendingly at meat-eaters. They are only deficient in education.

For absorption and proper use by the body, vitamin B_{12} also requires the action of certain microorganisms in your gut. These friendly bugs are destroyed by antibiotics. The most common cause of B_{12} deficiency is impaired absorption. So athletes who scoff antibiotics for every sniffle, or as "preventative" (God help us!), shouldn't be surprised if their red blood count is always down, and they have a permanent hitch in the giddy-up.

The 1995 adult RDI for vitamin B_{12} is 6.0 micrograms[1,2], ***triple*** the 1989 RDA of 2.0 micrograms.[3] This huge jump in adult requirements should tell you something about government recommendations. Research between 1989 and 1995 didn't uncover anything really new. But suddenly everyone needs triple the B_{12}.

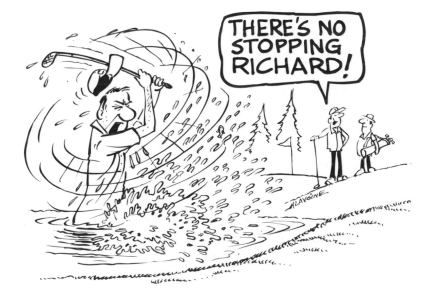

Cyanocobalamin For Athletes

Since I wrote **Optimum Sports Nutrition** in 1993, we have observed increasing vitamin B_{12} deficiency in athletes. Bruce Ames of the University of California, Berkeley has just reviewed the micronutrient status of Americans showing that up to 20% of the population do not eat even 50% of the RDA for vitamin B_{12}.[4] And a recent study of US national figure skaters show even lower intakes than the public.[5] Reanalyzing earlier studies in terms of the new RDI, most athletes surveyed under the old RDA standard would be classed as deficient, with vitamin B_{12} intake below 6 micrograms per day.[6,7]

For such an easy vitamin to get, it's a bit of a mystery that athletes don't get enough. Four possible causes that are easy to avoid are:

1. Excessively intense training (overtraining).

2. Poor quality vitamin B_{12} supplements.

3. Loss of B_{12} absorption due to destruction of symbiotic intestinal bacteria by antibiotic use or antibiotic residues in food.

4. Extreme dieting to lose bodyfat for aesthetic reasons, and to make weight to match the increasing number of weight categories in sports.

You can measure your B_{12} status in several ways. **Serum cobalamin** levels, determined by the *Lactobacillus leichmani* assay or **radioisotope dilution assay,** are reasonably reliable. A level above 250 pg/ml is acceptable for athletes.

That doesn't tell you anything about B_{12} absorption, however. For absorption you need the old and very cumbersome and expensive **urinary excretion of oral radio-labeled cobalamin** or **Schilling test**.[8] Using this test as a last resort, we have found some anemic athletes who have great difficulty absorbing vitamin B_{12}. Antibiotics use, which has destroyed their intestinal flora necessary for B_{12} absorption, is often the culprit.

A few athletes get regular B_{12} injections of 1000 times or more the RDA, and swear that it helps them. No evidence of toxicity but a pretty stupid practice. You get a bit of a buzz from the drug-like effect, then the body excretes 99.9% of it. The buzz may make you think you are performing better, but tests of B_{12} injections as ergogenics show zero improvement.[9]

The Colgan Institute uses daily oral supplements of 25 – 250 micrograms of cyanocobalamin. The majority of athletes will be well supplied at the lower end of this scale. The higher end will increase absorption by only 2 – 4 micrograms. But we have found quite a few athletes whose red blood cell count is better maintained with the higher intake. Toxicity of this range —nil.

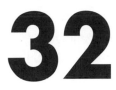

32

FOLATE, FOLIC ACID

Another of the eight vitamins of the B-complex so far identified by science, folate occurs in foods and in the human body in many chemical forms. It is essential for amino acid metabolism, manufacture of DNA, and all cell growth. Especially important to athletes, is folate's function in **erythropoiesis**, the formation of red blood cells. Folate is also essential for proper functioning of the brain, and for controlling body homocysteine levels, an excess of which damages your heart, your joints and especially your brain.[1]

Best food sources are fresh dark-green leafy vegetables, legumes and egg yolk. But folate levels vary widely in different samples of the same food[2] and food processing and storage now destroys about half the folate in the American diet,[3] and likely in the diets of most Westernized countries.

So it's not surprising that US National Academy of Science figures show that the folate content of even an excellent American diet has declined to only 280 – 300 micrograms per day.[3] And the latest surveys of Europe, just reported by de Bree and colleagues from

Wageningen University in Holland, show that average intakes of folate have fallen to 270 micrograms per day.[4] The latest National Diet and Nutrition Survey in Britain also reports widespread low intakes of folate.[5]

So, it's not surprising that excess levels of homocysteine have now become epidemic in Western Society, because research shows clearly that it takes at least 350 micrograms of folate per day to prevent this degenerative process, and about 800 micrograms per day to reverse it.[4,6]

Thereby hangs a sorry tale. When the US RDA Committee discovered in 1989 that the folate in the American diet had declined to an average of about 200 micrograms per day, they promptly cut the RDA for folate from 400 micrograms to 180-200 micrograms. Outrage by many scientists, including me, seemed to make little impression, until strong research showed that a simple folate supplement of 400 – 800 micrograms per day for pregnant women, prevents at least half the cases of spina bifida in newborns.[7] Government regulators promptly set the 1995 RDI back at 400 micrograms again.

We now know that following the RDA of 200 micrograms of folate per day also dramatically increases risk of colon cancer.[8] How many cases of spina bifida and colon cancer were caused by folk adhering to the RDA will never be known, but it's more than you and all your friends' fingers and toes! Makes you wonder whether the elevators of public health regulators ever get all the way to the top.

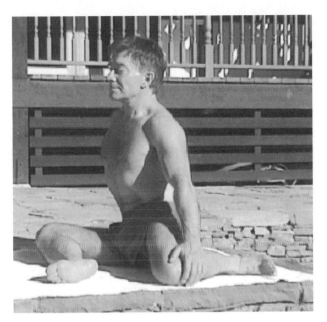

Michael Colgan demonstrating a piriformis stretch
from the Power Program.

Folate For Athletes

Folate requirements of athletes are unknown, but are likely to be much greater than those of sedentary people. In addition to its well-known functions in cell growth and amino acid metabolism, recent studies have shown that folate is involved in thousands of short-lived **folyl coenzyme** functions that cannot even be measured accurately with present technology.[9,10]

You can measure your own folate status fairly well using the **red-cell folate assay**. Don't use the serum folate assay: it's useless for athletes. Men in good condition that we have measured over the last two decades, almost all register red-cell folate levels above 200 ng/ml, and have total folate intakes from food and supplements above 600 micrograms per day.

Some research has reported that elite and club level athletes   consumed only 315 micrograms (male) and 200 micrograms (female) but did not measure their performance.[11] I'll bet it wasn't optimal. Other research is close to our findings, reporting folate intakes in   athletes of 510-630 micrograms per day.[12]

The Colgan Institute uses folic acid supplements of 400 – 2000 micrograms per day. Toxicity of this range —nil. Most athletes achieve apparently good red cell status of 200 ng/ml with 600 – 800 micrograms. But hold the press, because the multiple new functions of folic acid just discovered,[9,10] question the sufficiency of even this amount.

BIOTIN

One of the water-soluble B-complex, biotin forms part of two essential enzymes **pyruvate carboxylase** and **acetyl-coenzyme A carboxylase** involved in **gluconeogenesis**, (formation of glucose) and **lipogenesis**, (the formation of fatty acids). A third biotin-dependent enzyme is **3-methyl-crotonyl coenzyme A carboxylase**, essential for catabolism (breakdown) of branched chain amino acids.

Without biotin your body can't make proper use of fats, sugars or proteins. One of the first symptoms is falling hair. Then your skin and muscles disintegrate. And your brain, dependent on the long-chain fats manufactured from essential fats in the diet, starts to disintegrate too.[1]

If biotin is such serious stuff why don't we hear more about it in sports nutrition? I don't know. Research tends to go with what's new and hot for commercial exploitation. Biotin chemistry seemed to be known by the '70s. When large doses failed to restore balding heads, researchers lost interest. At that time they didn't appreciate the principle of synergy. If you want optimum performance, however, don't neglect biotin in your synergistic mix.

Best sources of biotin are liver, sardines, soy flour and egg yolk.[2] Don't use raw eggs in shakes or other foods though. Raw egg white contains a protein called **avidin** which binds biotin, so it is not bioavailable.[3] Cooking neutralizes the avidin.

US biotin intake is 28-42 micrograms/day.[2] Some biotin is also synthesized by microorganisms in the human gut, but no one knows how much. I hope that, by this point in the book, you get the picture that science still has a helluva lot to learn about vitamins.

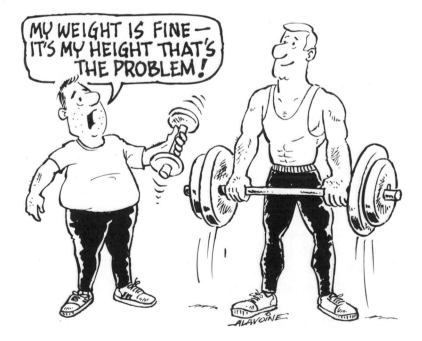

Biotin For Athletes

Biotin requirements are unknown. The 1980 US RDA Committee recommended 100-300 micrograms per day. But then they discovered that the average US diet contains only about 35 micrograms. So, in 1989 they quietly dropped the recommendation to 30-100 micrograms,[2] to satisfy food industry lobbyists who squeal like stuck pigs whenever evidence surfaces that their processed pap is inadequate. So much for science, yet numerous bowing and scraping health professionals still take RDA, and RDI and DRI pronouncements as gospel.

The range of biotin levels in whole blood taken from a representative sample of the US population is 215-750 pg/ml. Unfortunately, in order to be representative, a sample in America means people on poor nutrition who are likely to be sedentary, overweight, unfit, with some degree of atherosclerosis, joint degeneration and medication dependence. To apply the same standards to athletes is not exactly a mark of high intelligence. Nevertheless, some researchers have done so, and have found biotin levels "within normal ranges" in experienced athletes, and seem content.[4]

Never be content with existing science. Far from discovering almost everything, as the pretentious might posture, science is always scrabbling away on the edge of the unlimited. Our simian fingers and ponderous brains have hardly begun to unravel the mysteries of the human body. Now, in the supposedly enlightened 21st century we are still struggling just to measure biotin.[5] We are far from knowing how much is optimal for anyone.

At the Colgan Institute we measure serum biotin using the old, and not very accurate, ***Ochromonas danica*** assay. We take 1000 pg/ml and above as acceptable for athletes.   This level is easily achieved by supplementation with 600 – 5000 micrograms of biotin per day.   Most athletes seem to fare well near the lower end of this range.   Toxicity of range —nil.[2]

34

PANTOTHENIC ACID

Last of the eight vitamins that so far constitute the B-complex in science, pantothenic acid forms part of the multipurpose **coenzyme A** essential for breakdown of carbohydrates, fats and some proteins. It also forms part of one of the carrier proteins for the enzyme **fatty acid synthetase**, especially important for the manufacture of fats. Pantothenic acid is also essential for the manufacture of steroid hormones and brain neurotransmitters, and in the energy cycle.[1] So it's an important item for athletes.

Best food sources of pantothenic acid are meats, fish, whole grains and legumes. The richest food source is royal jelly, but it is also over 100 times more expensive than common foods. You can't get enough pantothenic acid from your diet. Average intake from food in the US is only 6 mg/day.[1] The 1995 RDI is 10 mg/day which puts most of the US population in deficit.

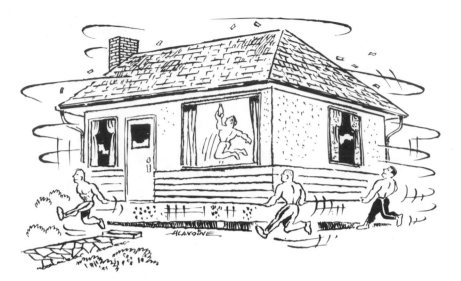

How many bodybuilders does it take to change a light builb?
Four: One to hold the bulb and three to rotate the building!

Pantothenic Acid For Athletes

Measurement of pantothenate is a representative sample of Americans, yields a whole blood reference range of 1120-1960 ng/ml.[2] As most of the population has deficient intake at the RDI level, presumably this range reflects pantothenate deficiency.

Athletes are even more deficient because pantothenate is released into the blood in large amounts during intense exercise and presumably used up.[3] Studies of elite athletes in a variety of sports, report that marathon runners and soccer players are below the reference range, and so are 30% of all athletes tested.[3]

As you might expect, silly short-term experiments using gram amounts of supplemental pantothenate show increases in blood levels[4,5] but, thankfully, no nonsensical "ergogenic" effects. Blood levels, however, increase for most substances used in mega-dose amounts, even water. Doesn't mean diddly.

I learned first-hand about pantothenate from its discoverer, the late Roger Williams of the University of Texas. Even then, 20-odd years ago, after 40 years of research, he knew it was a lot more complicated than the blasé accounts given in textbooks. Science still has no idea of the optimal amounts of pantothenate for athletes.

We used to measure status by the clumsy and time-consuming **24-hour urinary excretion of pantothenate,** taking 9 mg/day excretion or above as a measure of sufficiency. Our reasoning was that if your body is ditching the stuff in large amounts, you must be in excess. Now, I'm not so sure. Some athletes showing more than 9 mg/day urinary excretion of pantothenate still show classic symptoms of deficiency: insomnia, restlessness, burning feet, and loss of coordination. Trouble with "hotspots" in sports shoes is also a clue. If these symptoms are relieved by supplemental pantothenate, then the whole body was in bad biochemical disorder. You don't want to get to that stage with any nutrient.

Without a good standard to guide us, it makes sense to err on the plentiful side to assure good pantothenate nutrition. The Colgan Institute uses 20 - 200 mg/day supplemental pantothenate with athletes. Most will probably get enough near the bottom end of the range. Toxicity of range —nil.

"Fear does not exist
in any object or situation
It is constructed by you alone
A barrier to progress
Imposed solely by your mind."

- Michael Colgan
Program Your Mind Lecture Series, 2001

35

VITAMIN C ASCORBATES

Water-soluble vitamin C is not stored in the human body and must be eaten daily for optimal health. Traditional functions of vitamin C, from which the miniscule RDA and RDI were derived, mostly concern prevention of scurvy. This disease, exemplified by breakdown of skin and mucous membranes, occurs because vitamin C is essential for **hydroxylation of proline and lysine**. These two amino acids are required for manufacture of **collagen**, the tough, white, inelastic fibers of your skin, bones and connective tissues. About 50% of the structure of the cartilage pads that cushion your joints is collagen.

Later discovered functions of vitamin C include its role in manufacture of **carnitine**, required for the transport of fatty acids to the mitochondria of your cells for conversion to energy. Equally important, vitamin C is required for manufacture of your get-up-and-go brain neurotransmitters, **dopamine** and **norepinephrine**.

Latest discovered are the antioxidant functions of vitamin C. It is the major extracellular antioxidant in your body, and also functions at the cell membrane interface to regenerate fat-soluble vitamin E.

These functions may require gram amounts per day for optimal health.[1]

Best food sources of vitamin C are fruits and vegetables but amounts are highly variable.[2] Fresh red and green peppers and broccoli contain more than twice the vitamin C of the traditional orange. Oranges are a suspect source. Modern techniques of early picking, artificial ripening and storage all reduce vitamin C content. Strawberries, which cannot be stored for long, contain more vitamin C than oranges.[3]

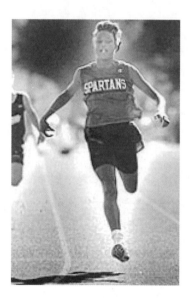

Marion Jones.
One of the fastest
women on Earth.

Vitamin C For Athletes

The medical literature contains many idiotic studies looking for short-term ergogenic effects of vitamin C. The same problem afflicts research on all the vitamins, but is especially prevalent in vitamin C research. So I want to use this work to expose the whole sad scenario, so that you can avoid being deceived by many, many vitamin studies, and their typical media and commercial distortions.

A huge stack of evidence shows beyond doubt that even marginal vitamin C deficiency impairs performance. Deficiency damages every part of your body by reducing manufacture of carnitine, thereby reducing availability of fat for energy, by reducing manufacture of brain neurotransmitters, by reducing collagen synthesis, and by exposing the whole body to the free radical damage caused by exercise.[1,4] Obviously a lot of athletes still don't know this research because studies commonly find that, overall, about 20% of all athletes in a wide variety of sports don't eat even the 1995 RDI of 60 mg of vitamin C.[5]

Some silly experiments and even sillier reviews of them may be to blame. There seems to be a common misconception, especially in the commercial vitamin community, that the controlled design of a double-blind crossover experiment excuses any sort of nonsense in its content. Double-blind means that neither subject nor researchers know which group of subjects is getting the real stuff, and which group is getting the placebo. And crossover means that both groups eventually get the real stuff.

In a typical gaff, researchers gave subjects 600 mg of vitamin C four hours before testing their grip strength, and found no effect.[6] Oh Lordy! Where do they think strength comes from? Out of the air! Strength increases as a result of resistance training which, over weeks and months causes your body to incorporate nutrients into new cells so as to build a better structure.

In another fiasco, researchers gave students undergoing sports training 1000 mg vitamin C for 21 days. They found no effects on VO_2 max or anaerobic performance.[7] Anyone who does research with students, knows well that their performance over 21 days is so variable, you have to use massive incentives to get any effect large enough to survive statistical analysis. No dinky little pill of vitamin C is going to do the job. Even then a "significant difference" is likely to be a result of faulty design or procedure.

A few studies claim to have found improvements in VO_2 max or reductions in oxygen debt with vitamin C supplementation over a few days. But when you examine the work in detail, it's easy to see how the effects could have been artifacts of the experimental design.[8] Fact is, it's almost impossible to measure true performance gains over a few weeks in the laboratory. All athletes know how variable their effort can be in the short-term, even in competition.

The only way to assess changes in performance properly is to measure the slope of improvement of an athlete's repeated performance over at least six months without supplementation, then over the same period with supplementation. If the slope of the two curves differs significantly, then you have something. An example from one of our studies is shown below.

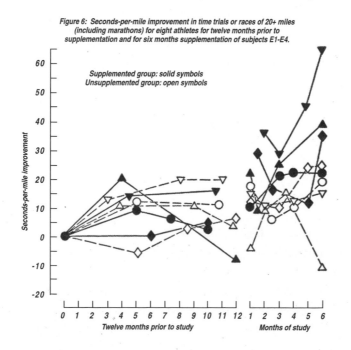

Figure 6: *Seconds-per-mile improvement in time trials or races of 20+ miles (including marathons) for eight athletes for twelve months prior to supplementation and for six months supplementation of subjects E1-E4.*

Measuring Changes In Biochemistry

The whole experimental situation changes if you are measuring discrete biochemical changes in the body rather than global performance. I'm pleased to see that the latest short-term research on vitamins is swinging that way.

We know, for example that exercise increases uncontrolled oxidation. In a typical recent study, measures of oxidative stress called **TBARS** (thiobarbituric-acid-reactive-substances) and **conjugated dienes**, were higher in athletes than control subjects. And ascorbic acid levels were lower in athletes than controls.[9] The athletes were using up their vitamin C like crazy.

It's clear that free radicals whack athletes' vitamin C, because other recent studies show that one gram of ascorbic acid reduces uncontrolled oxidation dramatically.[10,11] And new research shows reduced oxidation damage in athletes with vitamin C supplementation.[12,13]

Another good measure of vitamin C effects is upper respiratory tract infections (URTI). URTI are more common in athletics in intense training than in controls.[4,14] And vitamin C reduces them. In a representative study, Peters et al found that 1100 mg total vitamin C intake per day, substantially reduced URTI in ultramarathoners.[15]

Exercise-induced asthmatic symptoms are also common in athletes. Vitamin C stops them too. In a typical recent study, Cohen et al found that 2 grams supplemental vitamin C prevented bronchoconstriction very nicely.[16]

Measuring Vitamin C Status

Most studies on vitamin C status have used the old serum or plasma **2 – 6 – dichlorophenol – indophenol assay**, taking plasma ascorbic acid of 0.6 mg/dl as adequate. We used to use this assay, but recent evidence indicates it is too inaccurate. The level of plasma vitamin C achieved with any given amount of supplementation varies at least 3-fold in different individuals, so it isn't much of a guide to the vitamin C in their cells and organs.[17]

Better is the expensive **blood leucocyte ascorbate** determined by **high performance liquid chromatography (HPLC)**. Problem is, with all the new research on vitamin C suggesting that gram amounts per day are required to protect athletes in intense training from free radicals, we have no idea of the optimal level of ascorbic acid in leucocytes. Until there is a standard, we will continue to use large doses of ascorbic acid with athletes, 2 – 5 grams per day. Most will probably be well supplied near the lower end of this range. Toxicity of range – nil.

VITAMIN D CALCIFEROL

One of the many errors of 20th century attempts to define human nutrition, so-called "vitamin D" is not a vitamin at all. Your body can make it very well out of **dehydrocholesterol** in your skin and the **ultra-violet** in sunlight.[1] We continue to call it vitamin D, however, which doesn't say a lot for our smarts.

Vitamin D is a **prohormone**, one of the many groups of **sterols** used in the body which also occur in the food upon which we evolved.[1] It is essential for proper calcium, phosphorus and probably magnesium absorption and use in bones, muscle contraction, aerobic energy production, and immunity.[2]

The 1995 RDI for vitamin D is 10 micrograms. But vitamin labels still use the obsolete international units (I.U.). 10 micrograms = 400 IU. Because of fortification of milk and dairy foods with vitamin D to prevent **rickets**, most athletes probably get the RDI. Fish liver oil is also a potent source.

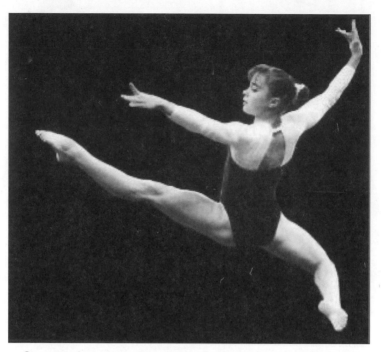

Gymnastics champion Lilya Podkopayeva in full flight.

Vitamin D For Athletes

No one knows how much vitamin D athletes need. What we do know is that intense endurance training lowers blood levels of **dihydrocholecalciferol**, the active form of vitamin D, for up to four weeks after training ceases.[3] Low blood vitamin D levels can cause muscle weakness and loss of calcium from bones. We suspect that vitamin D deficiency is involved in the female athlete triad syndrome, discussed ahead under vitamin K.

Exposure to 30 minutes of summer sunlight each day makes more vitamin D in your skin than the RDI. Sunblock, except the opaque kind, doesn't stop the process. Athletes who train outdoors in temperate or hot climates probably get plenty.

You can measure blood levels of **dihydrocholecalciferol** in a variety of ways but it doesn't mean much. Science has yet no normal range of vitamin D in blood that we can confidently apply to anyone. Vitamin D is fat-soluble and is stored in the body. Intakes of only five times the RDI (50 micrograms) may build up over long periods to be toxic, causing calcium deposits in soft tissues.[4] Unless you scoff vitamin D tablets or enjoy snacking on raw cod liver every day, you are unlikely to get an excess. The Colgan Institute uses 10 – 20 micrograms (400-800 IU) of supplemental vitamin D (cholecalciferol) daily with athletes.[3] Most seem well supplied at the lower end of this range. Toxicity of range – nil.

*"Form follows function.
You sit like a slug –
You grow like a slug."*

- Michael Colgan
Sports Lecture Series, 2002

37

VITAMIN E TOCOPHEROLS, TOCOTRIENOLS

Fat-soluble vitamin E consists of at least eight substances in food with differing forms and degrees of vitamin E activity in the body. Most active is the old standard 100% **d-alpha tocopherol** (now called in science **RRR-alpha-tocopherol**). Others, **d-beta-tocopherol** and **d-gamma-tocopherol** have about 50% and 10% activity respectively. More recently defined, **d-alpha tocotrienol** has about 30% and **d-beta tocotrienol** about 5% vitamin E activity.[1] Activity of the other forms of vitamin E is uncertain, but we do know that all eight act in synergy, and all are probably essential for optimal health.[1]

The primary function of vitamin E is antioxidant. The membranes of all cells in your body, especially your brain and nerves, are made of long-chain polyunsaturated fatty acids which are highly subject to attack by free radicals, or **reactive oxygen species (ROS)** as they are called in science nowadays.[1] Vitamin E is your major membrane protector, working in conjunction with the mineral selenium, vitamin C, coenzyme Q10 and glutathione.[1,2]

Even minor vitamin E deficiency is a big problem. My computer files contain more than 400 controlled studies showing that it causes neurological damage, loss of muscle function, erythrocyte hemolysis (red blood cells burst), damage to DNA, irreversible degeneration of the heart and organs, and increased risk of cardiovascular disease and certain cancers.[1-4]

I'm laying it out hot and heavy, because no one knows the amount of vitamin E required for optimal health. We just have not done the science yet. Nig-nog health professionals who quote the RDA (or newer recommendations derived from it) as sufficient, have probably never even read the RDA handbook and research papers. If they had, they would see that, using the amount of vitamin E in the American diet as a guide, the US National Research Council:

> "has established an arbitrary but practical allowance for male adults of 10 mg alpha-TEs per day. Because women are generally smaller, their allowance is 8 mg/day."[5]

Sounds like parents setting pocket-money for the kids, not an august scientific body determining the health of a nation. The 1995 RDI upped the ante to 30 alpha-TEs and dropped the gender discrimination. In terms of the obsolete IU standard still used on labels, 1 alpha-TE = 1 IU of the weak synthetic form of vitamin E, dl-alpha-tocopherol, and 0.67 IU of the natural-source vitamin E, d-alpha-tocopherol. So, depending on your source, 30 IU of vitamin E per day is supposed to suit everyone.

A ton of evidence shows that it takes many times that amount to inhibit cardiovascular disease, some cancers, decline of immune function, and oxidative damage caused by exercise.[1,6,7] Yet, primarily because of the lax government recommendation, thousands of uniformed health professionals purvey 30 IU as adequate, and seem to think it unimportant when surveys show that over two-thirds of the US population get less than even the old RDA of 10 IU.[8]

The best food sources of vitamin E are organic soybean oil, nuts and seeds, and whole grains. But being highly chemically active, much of the vitamin E in food is destroyed by storage and processing.[9] As the above surveys show, it's impossible to get sufficient vitamin E from food alone.

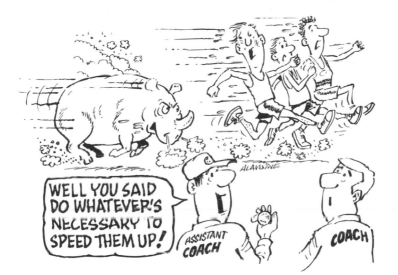

Vitamin E For Athletes

Throughout this book I present potent evidence that anyone who undertakes a sports training program requires greater nutrient intake than sedentary slugs. Vitamin E is a prime example. Insufficient vitamin E intake puts athletes' muscles, organs, blood cells and brain cells under increased oxidative stress, leading to injury and long-term illness. Any health professional who advises athletes that the RDA or RDI provide sufficient vitamin E, is guilty of malpractice.

Numerous studies still measure vitamin E levels in blood. Pretty well useless, because vitamin E is carried in your blood by lipoproteins, so the level found depends greatly on lipoprotein levels.[10] For a given vitamin E intake, unhealthy folk with high LDL levels, will show much higher vitamin E than athletes with healthy lipid profiles. The best test for deficiency in reference to average public levels, is **stability of erythrocytes in hydrogen peroxide**.[11] As yet we have no test of sufficiency.

Until we have better measures, the Colgan Institute uses supplements of vitamin E with athletes that reflect the research showing reductions in oxidative stress and improved muscle repair. We use only natural-source vitamin E (d-alpha-tocopheryl succinate) in amounts of 400 – 1600 mg per day plus mixed tocopherols and tocotrienols of 400 – 800 mg, yielding approximately 700 – 2600 alpha-TE or IU. Most athletes are well supplied near the bottom of this range. Toxicity of range —nil.[12]

38

VITAMIN K

Last of the fat soluble vitamins yet discovered, vitamin K comes in three chemical forms, **phylloquinone**, the active form in the body, which also occurs in foods, **menaquinone**, which is manufactured by flora in your gut, and the inactive synthetic form **menadione**, used for vitamin K supplements, which, hopefully, is converted to phylloquinone in the body. Vitamin K functions in blood clotting and, in conjunction with vitamin D, in regulation of bone formation.[1] If you want strong, athletic bones, better get enough K.

Best food sources are fresh, green leafy vegetables. But sources are highly variable, providing 50 – 800 micrograms of vitamin K per 100 grams.[2] The **SAD** (Standard American Diet) contains 300-500 micrograms of vitamin K per day. The three pounds (1.4 kilos) or so of flora in your gut also make vitamin K, assumed to be about the same amount again.[3] But microbiological synthesis of vitamin K in the gut is also highly variable, depending on your intestinal health. Antibiotics for example, wipe out the process entirely.

The 1995 RDI for vitamin K is 80 micrograms, same as the old RDA.[2] By this standard, populations of Westernized countries should be getting plenty. It is pretty obvious, however, to anyone who takes off the blinders, that a lot of folk are seriously deficient in vitamin K.

Here's how it goes. The RDI is based solely on the vitamin K required to maintain "normal" blood clotting, estimated at an average of 45 micrograms per day for men and 35 micrograms for women. By this measure, the RDI of 80 micrograms should cover everyone. And the bottom of the range of estimated daily vitamin K in the US of 300 micrograms from food, plus 300 micrograms made in the gut, should be way more than necessary. Why then are more than 50% of US infants deficient in vitamin K the day they are born, many requiring massive supplementation to prevent them bleeding to death?[3,4]

New-borns get all their vitamin K from mother's milk, because their intestines are not yet colonized with vitamin K synthesizing bacteria. Thus, many mothers must be vitamin K deficient because the milk is not supplying enough.[8,3] So, whatever vitamin K mothers are getting in food and microbiological synthesis today must be insufficient also. It could not have been this way in evolution, otherwise humanity would not have survived.

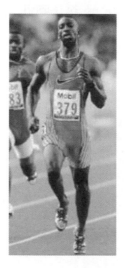

**Michael Johonson
at full speed.**

Vitamin K For Athletes

By now you may be wondering what the hell has all the above to do with athletes. Let me explain by way of example. A serious problem of female athletes has recently become so prevalent, it is now called "**the female athlete triad**" in medical literature.[5-7] It consists of restricted eating to minimize bodyfat, loss of menstruation caused by intense training, and loss of bone density.[5-7] Severe cases are often cruelly called "double A – O" that is anorexia, amenorrhea, and osteoporosis. (or osteopenia, reduced bone mass).

This triad causes severe disruption of the hormonal cascade by affecting the hypothalamus and pituitary in the brain and also the adrenal glands. Bone growth is severely retarded – irreversibly in many young female athletes.[5-8] Affected athletes, and there are many of them, also suffer a higher incidence of stress fractures, scoliosis, and musculoskeletal injuries associated with weak bones.[7-10] Later in life they are also at high risk of the horrors of osteoporosis.[11] We have studied this problem intensively at the Colgan Institute, and are now pretty sure that insufficient structural nutrients in the diet is the major cause. The primary deficiencies seem to be calcium, vitamin D and vitamin K.

Unfortunately, the work is not known well enough yet in sports medicine. Nutritional attempts to correct the female athlete triad usually consist only of calcium supplements.[12] But the evidence is starting to get out there. In one recent study, Cracium et al at Masstricht University in Holland measured the vitamin K status of amenorrheic athletes, using the **calcium binding capacity** of the bone protein **osteocalcin** circulating in their blood. Osteocalcin is essential to bone formation and is vitamin K dependent. The athletes were all vitamin K deficient. They were then supplemented for one year with 10 mg vitamin K per day, over 100 times the RDI. Bone formation increased by 15 – 20%.[13]

All coaches and health professionals working with athletes should study this research carefully. A simple nutrient supplement could save a great deal of misery and disease. And don't think that males are immune. Their deficiency may not show as blatantly as amenorrhea, but the **calcium binding capacity of blood osteocalcin assay** may tell a different story. And the calcium assay covered in the next chapter will help too. As I noted earlier, vitamin D sufficiency is unknown, but case studies we have done adding vitamin D to vitamin K and calcium have shown the greatest improvement.

At the Colgan Institute we use 200 – 1000 mcg of menadione with athletes. Most males are probably well served in the lower half of this range, most females in the upper half. Menadione can be toxic in large amounts, but we have found no reports nor had any cases of toxicity with this range.

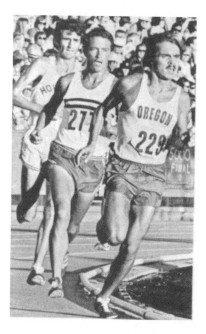

*The late great
Steve Prefontaine
killing the
competition with his
iron will.*

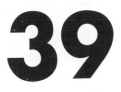

TESTING VITAMIN STATUS

For athletes and coaches who want to assess their vitamin status, below is a summary of the tests noted in the previous vitamin chapters. These are the tests we have found helpful while not outrageously expensive. Latest science indicates, however, that numerous vitamins have functions that were previously unknown, and that exercise uses more vitamins than previously thought. So it is unlikely that definitive tests yet exist for any of them.

Also, tests using blood or urine are really measuring only the transport of vitamins, not their use in tissues and organs. And we now know that different tissues and organs may use greatly differing amounts of each vitamin.

If we have learned anything from the arrogant blundering of nutrition science in the 20th century, we should all be bowing deep before the chemical miracles of human bodies, and grass and trees, in respectful acknowledgement that Nature made all the locks and still hides most of the keys.

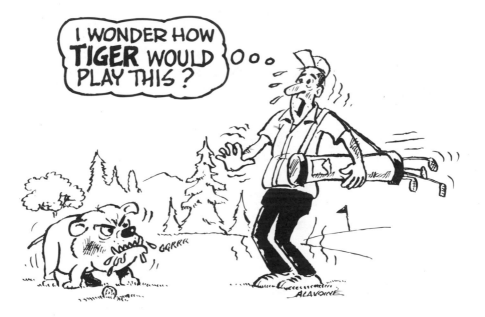

Biochemical Tests Used With Athletes

Vitamin	Test	Acceptable Status
A	Serum retinol	Above 40 mcg/dl
B$_1$	Erythrocyte TLPP	Below 10% TLPP Stimulation
B$_2$	EGRAC	Above 1.35
B$_3$	Urine N-methylnicotinamide	Above 3.0 mg/gram creatine
B$_6$	EGOT	Below 1.25
B$_{12}$	Serum cobalamin*	Above 250 pg/ml
Folate	Erythrocyte folate	Above 200 ng/ml
Biotin	Serum biotin*	Above 1000 pg/ml
Pantothenic Acid	24 hour urinary excretion*	Above 9 mg/day
C	Plasma 2 - 6 - dichlorophenol-indopehnol*	Above 0.6 mg/dl
D	No acceptable test	
E	For deficiency only. erythrocyte stability in hydrogen peroxide	Different labsl have differing assay ranges
K	Calcium-binding capacity of osteocalcin	Different labsl have differing assay ranges

* Tests starred are commonly used but somewhat doubtful in validity and reliability
© Copyright: Colgan Institute, 2000

"Like the grope and groan therapies before them, the consciousness-raising therapies of today represent extreme excursions of the tendency of our culture to evade, distort and vulgarize our humanity, seeking to produce spontaneity by artifice, to provide access to experiential knowledge by reducing it to a commodity, to engineer autonomy by group pressure."

- Michael Colgan
Program Your Mind Lecture Series, 2001

ACETYL-L-CARNITINE

To boost your anabolic drive to gain muscle and strength, you have to do everything possible to maximize function of the neurotransmitter systems of the striatal cortex and hypothalamus. These are the parts of your brain that control hormone release from the pituitary gland. In my book *Hormonal Health*, I show how they do this mainly through the activity of two neurotransmitters, acetylcholine and dopamine. One potent strategy to boost their activity is to increase the amount of acetyl-L-carnitine in your brain.

The natural amino acid L-carnitine occurs throughout your body and in many foods, including milk.[1] But you can't use L-carnitine supplements. To affect your brain, supplements have to be in the acetylated form in order to pass easily through the blood-brain barrier. Once it gets into the brain, acetyl-L-carnitine performs miracles.

I have space to cite only a couple of examples from the pile of more than 100 studies on my desk showing that acetyl-L-carnitine protects the brain in multiple ways.[2-4] It is an antioxidant that prevents perioxidation of brain lipids.[5] That is, it prevents your brain, which is mostly made of fat from going rancid. In turn this action reduces the build-up of **lipofuscin** (brown fats), cellular debris that interferes with brain function.[6] This non-toxic compound is so powerful, it even protects your optic nerves from aging.[4]

Protecting the visual system is particularly pertinent to humans, because failing vision is a prominent characteristic of human life after age 30. No controlled studies have yet been done on normal humans to see if acetyl-L-carnitine will help. In diabetics, however, acetyl-L-carnitine is being used with some success to inhibit the retinal damage and vision loss common to this disease.[7]

In individual case studies at the Colgan Institute, we also have a number of reports of improved vision in folk who regularly take acetyl-L-carnitine. By improved, I mean that their optometrists have had to reduce the power of their glasses and contact lenses.

The Acetylcholine Connection

From animal studies, we know that acetyl-L-carnitine supplements increase an enzyme called acetylcoenzyme A. This enzyme supports the acetylcholine system in the striatal cortex and hypothalamus, by providing material for another chemical, carnitine-acetyltransferase, that is essential to acetylcholine production.[8] All the current animal evidence indicates that acetyl-L-carnitine increases brain acetylcholine.

Healthy humans object to their brains being diced and sliced, so the human evidence is indirect. Nevertheless, carnitine-acetyltransferase is very low in the brains of folk who die from Alzheimer's and other forms of senility.[9] And senility is closely linked with degeneration of the hippocampus in the striatal cortex. If acetyl-L-carnitine benefits acetylcholine metabolism in humans, it should help Alzheimer's as well as eyes.

It does. Multiple studies show large improvements in Alzheimers and other senile patients supplemented with acetyl-L-carnitine.[10,11] One of the most recent, was done by Dr. Jay Pettigrew and colleagues at the University of Pittsburgh Medical School. They found that Alzheimers patients given acetyl-L-carnitine for a year, showed far less mental deterioration than a control group. Measures of brain function, using nuclear magnetic resonance, also showed less deterioration in the patients' brains than in the brains of controls.[10]

Effects are even more potent with mildly senile patients. A multi-center controlled trial in Italy, gave 500 patients a moderate supplement of 1500 mg of acetyl-L-carnitine per day for 90 days. Even in that short period, they showed significant improvements in intelligence, memory, and emotions. These effects persisted when tested again a month after supplementation ceased. Acetyl-L-carnitine will improve brain function even in brains that have been allowed to deteriorate beyond permanent repair. Taken before irreversible brain damage occurs, it can work wonders.

In a representative example highly pertinent to athletes, healthy men and women aged 22-27 were supplemented with moderate doses of acetyl-L-carnitine for 30 days. Complex video game tests before and after supplementation showed big improvements in speed of learning, speed of reaction, and reduction of errors. This simple amino does more than just protect the brain, it may also improve normal cognition.[12]

Acetyl-L-Carnitine Also Boosts Dopamine

Because of its clear chemical connection to acetylcholine, not much research has been done yet, on effects of acetyl-L-carnitine on dopamine, the second major neurotransmitter that controls your hormone cascade. Animal studies now show that acetyl-L-carnitine benefits dopamine directly.

Researchers at the Nathan Kline Institute in Orangeburg, New York, examined effects of acetyl-L-carnitine on dopamine release in the striatal cortex. They found that aged mice, given acetyl-L-carnitine for three months, showed much improved dopamine activity, despite an age-related loss of about half of their dopamine receptors.[13]

The Kline Institute study was for only three months, and the aged animals used had already suffered a lot of irreversible cell death in their brains before it began. Studies using supplementation for longer periods, show that acetyl-L-carnitine can prevent much of the brain cell loss of usual aging if begun early enough. It inhibits cell loss not only in the striatal cortex, but also in the **prefrontal cortex**, your primary area for cognition, and in the **occipital cortex**, the brain area at the back of your head that is primary for vision.[14] If you start early, acetyl-L-carnitine may protect not only your anabolic drive, but also other crucial parts of your brain.

The Cortisol Link

If acetyl-L-carnitine helps maintain dopamine and acetylcholine metabolism, you would expect that it also acts as an anticatabolic. Why? Because when the neurotransmitters in the striatal cortex are working well, they help to keep **cortisol** under control. Cortisol, commonly known as the stress hormone, is highly catabolic to muscle.

No human studies yet, but animal studies do show greatly reduced cortisol levels in animals subjected to stress, when they are supplemented with acetyl-L-carnitine.[2] It's a good bet it will work on humans in the same way.

Dosage and Timing

No one knows exactly how much acetyl-L-carnitine to use. Most studies have been done with 500-2500 mg per day. At the Colgan Institute we use 500-2000 mg, taken in the morning on rising. That's the best regime we know to synchronize the brain stimulation caused by acetyl-L-carnitine, with the rest of the hormone cascade.

Some researchers suggest the taking acetyl-L-carnitine in the evening, because of the large release of hormones during sleep. Not a good idea. By stimulating the excitatory neurotransmitters acetyl-choline and dopamine, acetyl-L-carnitine makes them dominant over the activity of the neurotransmitter **serotonin**. In your circadian rhythm, serotonin activity naturally becomes dominant at night and promotes sleep. Serotonin is also the base material from which your pineal gland makes melatonin. It's likely that acetyl-L-carnitine taken later than 3:00-4:00pm suppresses normal serotonin and melatonin activity, and disrupts both the hormone cascade and your sleep cycle.

No controlled trials have shown this action yet, but you can test it yourself. Taking a good dose of acetyl-L-carnitine at night, should convince you in one try. After ten hours of itchy, twitchy insomnia, your morning mirror reveals eyes like holes burned in a blanket, over a mouth that mutters repeatedly, "Never, never, never again."

Used in the right way, however, acetyl-L-carnitine is a great boon to both your brain and your anabolic drive. But you have to begin early, while most of your brain cells are still alive and kicking.

"We have become an obtuse culture which trusts its morality to TV evangelists, its justice to politicions, and its arts to entrepreneurs."

- Michael Colgan
Program Your Mind Lecture Series, 2002

41

PHOSPHATIDYL-SERINE

In your brain cell membranes, some essential fatty acids are arranged in a configuration called phosphatidylserine, a mixture of phosphorus and fat, mostly fat. Phosphatidylserine oversees a multitude of tasks. It stimulates release of brain neurotransmitters, it activates transport of nutrients, and it regulates glucose availability. Much of the brain activity involved in memory and learning is dependent on continuous adequate levels of phosphatidylserine.[1,2]

Phosphatidylserine levels decline with usual aging. After age 25, you are on the downward slope. Some researchers suggest that this decline underlies the increasing difficulty of learning new material as you age.[3,4]

In May 1981, I and my labmates ran around Rockefeller University shouting "Eureka." We had just received new Italian research, showing that a supplemental form of phosphatidylserine improved memory and learning in aged rats. A pristine memory, and the ability to learn rapidly, are the pearls of a researcher's existence. Even back then, 21 years ago, we knew that all the nutrition, all the supplements, all the exercise, come to naught unless you can protect the functions of your brain cell membranes. Surrounded by doddery old professors, who demonstrated every day that they had lost the ability to think, we were very aware of our own mortality.

At that time, the phosphatidylserine was being laboriously extracted from cow brains and cost a bundle. Nevertheless, we were determined to get enough for research, and for ourselves. Right on the brink of bankrupting our research grants, the bad news broke. Despite spectacular results in rejuvenation of brain function, some of the rats were dying of **spongiform encephalopathy**. Some batches of the phosphatidylserine were carrying a stowaway, a slow virus that causes "mad cow disease." That was the end of that.

In 1990 the whole picture changed. The Lipogen company succeeded in making vegetable phosphatidylserine from Savoy cabbages and soy lecithin. By 1992, they were manufacturing a commercial product that was both inexpensive and completely safe. We were back in business to save our membranes.

To date there are only animal studies with the vegetable compound, though bovine phosphatidylserine has improved brain function in numerous studies of human senility.[5-8] In a representative test of the vegetable compound, baby mice were given phosphatidylserine from birth to sixty days old, and compared with a control group. At one month, the supplemented mice showed higher intelligence than control mice. At two months, the supplemented mice learned faster and more accurately than adult mice.[9] After a quarter century of research, I think the evidence is now sufficient to warrant addition of at least 100 mg of vegetable phosphatidylserine to your daily supplement mix.

MELATONIN

Media reports applaud melatonin as a natural sleeping pill, and a way to beat jet lag. True enough, but these are only minor reflections of its functions. We know now that deficiency of pineal melatonin disrupts your hormones, your cognition, your immune system and your emotions. Melatonin deficit also increases your risks of cancer, cardiovascular disease, senility and a host of other disorders. When your melatonin runs down, everything goes.

I can't cover the mass of new studies here, but if you doubt me, Dr. Russell Reiter, Professor of Neuroendocrinology at The University of Texas, San Antonio, has published an easy-reading, 250-page summary of the evidence.[1] That should be enough to convince you.

The Aging Clock

What you need to know here, is that pineal output of melatonin declines rapidly with usual aging. This decline is so reliable that numerous researchers now refer to the pineal gland as "The Aging Clock."[2]

I constructed the figure below from an average of all the major studies. In your mid-twenties peak nighttime melatonin output is about 50pg/ml. By age 30 it declines to 40pg/ml. By age 50 it drops to less than half the youthful level. By age 70, it's down to 10pg/ml, only 20% of the melatonin you have in your twenties. That's one reason a lot of old folk don't sleep well: they have insufficient melatonin.[2]

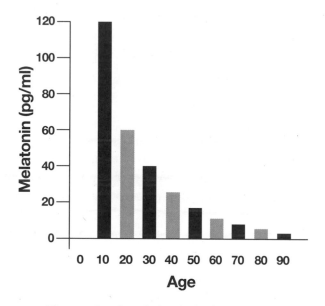

Nocturnal melatonin levels decline with usual aging.
Source: Colgan Institute, San Diego, CA, 1998.

The first thing to do to maintain the function of your whole hormonal system, is to restore the melatonin output of the master controller - the pineal gland. Without sufficient melatonin to direct the synchrony of your other hormones, you have little chance of keeping them in balance.

Most dangerous are the end-organ hormones at the bottom of the cascade, androgens and estrogens. They act directly on tissue to cause growth, therefore require the greatest control. With much of the current stimulation of the hormone cascade by athletes, and the huge practice of illicit hormone use, that vital control is non-existent. Many physicians, for example, will prescribe testosterone to masters athletes to bring their testosterone up to youthful levels, without restoring melatonin or any of the other controllers further upstream. By doing so, they are putting in a powerful growth chemical with freedom to run wild. No surprise that it eventually causes enough wild growth to turn to cancer.

Benefits Of Melatonin Replacement

Besides maintaining and restoring the circadian synchrony of your hormones, many new studies show further benefits of melatonin. First, it is a powerful brain antioxidant that inhibits brain aging by destroying free radicals. These are damaging oxidation chemicals that are produced by toxins such as alcohol, and by normal brain metabolism of oxygen.[3]

Melatonin may also act as a bodily antioxidant to prevent cancer.[4] It also boosts immunity against numerous other diseases, including AIDS.[2] It also helps to lower cholesterol and protect your heart.[2] It gives you better sleep and rest,[5] and it slows the decline in growth hormone that occurs with usual aging after 20 years of age.[6]

Nutritional Melatonin

If you can't abide the thought of taking nightly pills, you can go for night-time snacks of foods that are high in melatonin. Best sources are slow-cooking rolled oats, whole brown rice, and sweet corn, which contain 20-50mcg of melatonin per ounce. Bananas and tomatoes contain about half as much. Studies report that feeding animals such high melatonin foods increases their melatonin levels.[2]

Supplementing your diet with 500-1000mg of calcium also increases melatonin levels.[2] You should have at least this amount in your daily multi-vitamin/mineral. It has a larger effect on melatonin production when taken at night.

Vitamins B[3] (niacin) and B[6] (pyridoxine) affect melatonin too.[7] Other B vitamins and other essential nutrients are also likely to have a hand in the process, because all vitamins and minerals work in synergy with each other.[8,9] But the studies have not yet been done. Until scientists have had time to document the precise interactions, a *complete* multi-vitamin/mineral supplement provide sensible nutrition insurance for melatonin maintenance.

Dose And Timing

Taking melatonin in a sublingual pill is the best way. It's not expensive. Nor do you need much. No one knows the ideal dose, but 1.0 - 12.0 mg per night covers most people. I personally take 3 mg, which seems sufficient to peak my nighttime melatonin levels near those of an average 25-year-old. My colleagues and clients take anywhere from 0.5 mg to 15.0 mg. In 14 years of using melatonin in these doses, we have no reports of side-effects.

By usual toxicological tests, toxicity of melatonin is extremely low. Even doses of several hundred milligrams produce nothing more than sleepiness.[2] But no one knows the invisible long-term effects of large doses, subtle effects that may interfere with bodily processes. We know that excess melatonin can disrupt the hormone cascade, because very high doses make a reliable contraceptive.[2] For maintenance purposes, a few milligrams per night is plenty.

Timing is essential to avoid disrupting the synchrony of the hormone cascade. We take melatonin so that its presence in the bloodstream will coincide as far as possible with the natural nocturnal burst of the hormone. This burst occurs from about 1 am to 4 am in folk who keep usual sleep hours.[2] Western Society generally goes to bed around 10:30 pm or 11:30 pm, depending on which TV news is least offensive. To allow for digestion and entry into the brain, we take melatonin right before accustomed bedtime.

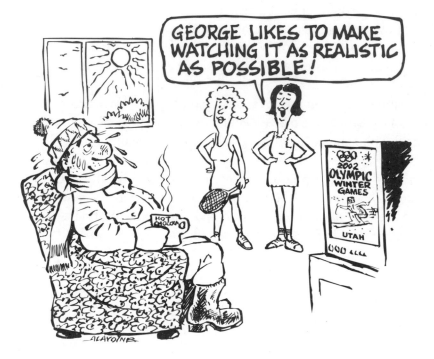

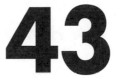

43

S-ADENOSYL-METHIONINE

Rare in the past, over the last 40 years elevated homocysteine in the blood has become a common condition, now affecting many millions of people in Western Society. It is yet another telling example of human creation of disease, by the destruction of the essential nutrients in our food, and the adoption of lifestyles that fail to provide sufficient amounts of the structural materials required to maintain the human body.

Most folk now know of Dr. Kilmer McCully's research showing that elevated homocysteine is a strong risk factor for cardiovascular disease. In February 1998, in a guest editorial in the Journal of the American Medical Association, McCully recounts the long road he traveled to achieve medical acceptance, The same issue details the research that vindicates his 30 years of patient work.[1,2] Little did he know that he was also pioneering a route to the prevention and cure of joint and soft tissue injuries in athletes.

How Homocysteine Rises

We know from McCully's work, and from the research of hundreds of scientists who now collaborate with him, exactly which essential structural materials are missing from our diets, that allow homocysteine to rise - folic acid and vitamin B_{12}. A quick peek at the chemistry reveals all. Homocysteine is a normal component of your body, an intermediate in the orchestrated symphony of biochemical events that keep you healthy. Folic acid, vitamin B_{12}, (and probably vitamin B_6) all act in concert to prevent homocysteine from rising to toxic levels by converting it back to the non-toxic essential amino acid methionine.[1-9] The basic cycle is shown below.

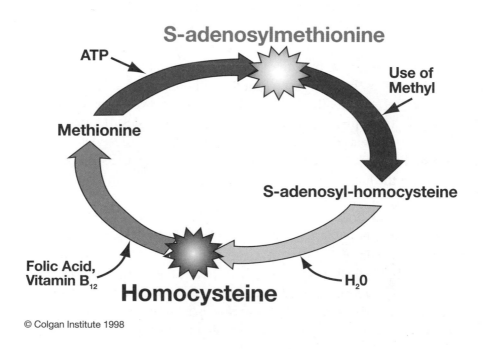

© Colgan Institute 1998

Figure 3:
The SAMe/Homocysteine Cycle

This chemistry is intimately connected with the metabolism of S-adenosyl-methionine - SAMe. SAMe is the activated form of methionine used by almost every cell of your body in what are called **methylation reactions**. If the body is short of folic acid, and vitamin B_{12}, then a lot of your methionine gets tied up as elevated homocysteine, reducing the amount available for the body to make a normal level of SAMe.[1-9]

Even a slight or intermittent deficiency of vitamin B_{12} and folic acid, if continued over years, allows homocysteine levels to gradually rise and SAMe levels to gradually fall.[3-9] Because many athletes, especially strength athletes, focus on protein and low-glycemic grains as their main diet, and neglect fresh vegetables, we thought they might be short on folic acid and B_{12}. So we did a quick sampling of strength athletes who suffered a lot of joint and soft tissue problems, and measured their homocysteine levels. On average they showed low intakes of folic acid and elevated levels of homocysteine compared to non-athlete controls.

Folic Acid, & Vitamin B12 Deficiencies Rampant

It certainly supports our finding on a few cases if folic acid and vitamin B_{12} deficiencies are widespread in Western Society, and these deficiencies are linked with high homocysteine levels. The latest review of studies of folic acid intake in Europe, was published recently by Dr. A de Bree and colleagues at the Department of Human Nutrition of Wageningen University in Holland. Mean dietary intake of folic acid is only 291 mcg per day for men and 247 mcg per day for women. This is woefully insufficient to prevent a toxic increase in homocysteine. As these researchers indicate, to keep homocysteine at healthy levels requires a **minimal** daily intake of 350 mcg of folic acid.[10]

Similar low folic acid intake is widespread in the U.S. where the folate content of a good diet is only 280-300 mcg and the average daily intake is a lot less than that.[11] The folic acid intake in America has declined in line with the degradation of our food to such an extent, that the previous RDA of 400 mcg was reduced to 200 mcg to suit, as that is all you get in an average American diet. No surprise then that homocysteine levels are high and rising, despite continuing recommendations from various health authorities that the public should have a minimum folic acid intake of 400 mcg per day.[3-9]

In Britain also, the recent National Diet and Nutrition Survey (1997), reports widespread low intake of folic acid and vitamin B_{12}, strongly correlated with high homocysteine levels. Researchers there conclude that the link between homocysteine and vitamin deficiency is so strong, that plasma homocysteine be used as one measure of folic acid and vitamin B_{12} status in the British population.[12] And leading researchers in Europe and America, also concur that high plasma homocysteine is a reliable marker of both folate and vitamin B_{12} deficiencies.[2,12]

Homocysteine Hurts Your Joints

There are no studies yet of homocysteine and joint and soft tissue injuries in athletes. But we can get some clues from studies of arthritic joint degeneration. A representative study of homocysteine and rheumatoid arthritis, by Dr. R Roubinoff and colleagues at Tufts University in Boston, Massachusetts reports that nearly half of all rheumatoid patients tested showed folic acid deficiency, and a high proportion showed vitamin B_{12} deficiency. **All** the patients showed elevated homocysteine. Their blood homocysteine levels were 33% higher than healthy hospital workers used as controls.[6]

In arthritic forms of fibromyalgia and chronic fatigue, a new study of women patients has been published by Dr. B Regland and team at the Institute of Clinical Neuroscience of Göteborg University in Sweden. They found that **every one** of these women had elevated homocysteine levels in their cerebrospinal fluid.[3]

High Homocysteine/Low SAMe Damages Your Brain

If you don't care about your joints, or don't have joint problems, you might still like to protect your smarts. High homocysteine whacks your brain, bad. The latest review of studies of older people worldwide, has just been completed at the Department of Clinical Medicine of Perugia University in Italy by Dr. L Parnetti and colleagues. The data reveal that low intakes of folic acid and vitamin B_{12}, and consequent high homocysteine and low SAMe, are accompanied by depression and dementia.[1]

A similar review of the controlled studies of people of all ages was published in 1997 by Dr. T Bottiglieri and group from the Institute of Metabolic Diseases of Baylor University Medical Center in Dallas, Texas. They found that folic acid and vitamin B_{12} deficiency, and consequent elevated homocysteine, cause depression and dementia, and also damage the myelin sheaths that protect the nerves in your brain.[8]

High brain homocysteine also causes high production of **homocysteic acid** in the brain, known to cause excessive brain stimulation and cognitive disturbance.[4] Worse, high brain homocysteine causes **microangiopathy** (micro-strokes), damaging small blood vessels, with resulting permanent mental impairment.[13] Basically, if you have high homocysteine levels, you are one big mess.

Folate, B₁₂ And SAMe Reduce Homocysteine

The next step on our path to beat joint and soft tissue injuries, is to examine whether vitamins can reduce homocysteine levels, and whether SAMe is a useful addition to this treatment. In 1997, Dr. M Ward and team at the University of Ulster in Ireland, confirms earlier work on folate supplementation. They show unequivocally that 400 mcg per day of folic acid reliably reduces homocysteine levels.[14]

The latest representative study, published in the New England Journal of Medicine in April 1998 by Dr. M Malinow and colleagues, gave patients with coronary artery disease a breakfast cereal fortified with folic acid. Fortification with 499 mcg and 655 mcg of folic acid per day raised plasma folic acid by 65% and 106% respectively, and reduced homocysteine levels by 11% and 14%.[15]   From this and similar studies, the Colgan Institute has derived a dose of 1200 mcg per day of folic acid as appropriate for athletes with joint problems and elevated homocysteine levels.

After reviewing 35 recent studies, Dr. M Moghadasian and colleagues at St. Paul's Hospital in Vancouver, Canada recommend that vitamin B_{12} and folic acid be used together to lower homocysteine levels.[16]   It's sensible to always include vitamin B_{12} in a supplementation regimen, for two reasons. First, vitamin B12 is required for the SAMe/homocysteine cycle. Second, some folk have a vitamin B_{12} deficiency, which would be masked by folic acid supplementation alone, and would continue to progressively damage the body.[17]   From all controlled studies to date, the Colgan Institute has derived a dose of vitamin B_{12} of 100 mcg per day as both safe and effective.

SAMe Lowers Homocysteine

SAMe works too. A new study has just been published by Dr. F Loehrer and colleagues at University Children's Hospital in Basel, Switzerland. They show that, even in healthy subjects, 400 mg of SAMe per day improves folic acid metabolism and reduces homocysteine levels.[18] At the Colgan Institute we use a minimum of 400 mg of SAMe per day for athletes with joint problems.

Combined with glucosamine sulfate and chondroitin sulfate covered in chapters ahead, and essential fats covered in Volume 2, SAMe plus folic acid and vitamin B_{12} provide the best strategy we know to maintain those pesky joints.

44

CREATINE

Adenosine triphosphate (ATP) *stored* in your muscles is the only fuel instantly available for energy. Stored ATP is therefore the only fuel capable of generating 100% muscle contraction. Once stored ATP is exhausted, other fuels dominate the energy supply. Because all of them must be converted to ATP before they can be used, available energy per second declines, so maximum muscle contraction declines, also.

You can store enough ATP for about 4-5 seconds of maximum contraction, enough to do a 1-rep max squat, throw a javelin, or run 50 meters. As 100-meter sprinters know only too well, maximum muscle contraction cannot be maintained beyond about 5 seconds. After that the goal is to lose as little speed as possible until you pass the finish line.

Because it is the only way you can ever put maximum load on your muscles, muscle contraction by stored ATP is unquestionably the most effective for building strength. It creates the most extensive micro-damage, which then triggers the greatest adaptive muscle growth[1].

Unfortunately, it's also the most dangerous way to train, because, at 100% contraction, the muscle and its attachments are at greatest risk. That's why folk who are constantly pushing the max, track & field athletes, powerlifters, weightlifters, and professional athletes are always on the knife edge of muscle and connective tissue injury.

The Creatine System

After 4-5 seconds of maximum exercise, creatine phosphate (CP) becomes the dominant energy control, permitting *near* maximum muscle contraction for another 5-6 seconds, a total of 10-11 seconds. That's enough to do a 4-rep set or sprint the 100 meters. This ATP/CP interaction is also anaerobic, and uses no glycogen, glucose, fatty acids or amino acids.

Because the ATP/CP system cannot permit maximum contraction, muscle is at less risk, so this level of exercise is much safer. Yet it still generates substantial micro-trauma, which, in turn, triggers near maximum growth. Overall, the ATP/CP 10-second window of exercise, provides the best combination of safety and efficacy for optimum strength training. That's why creatine is important to athletes.

How Creatine Works

Though ATP is the life force of all living things, it's just a simple chemical, a molecule of adenosine bonded to three molecules of phosphate. By a process still completely unknown to science, a command from your nervous ststem to contract a muscle, breaks one of these phosphate bonds, causing a chemical release of energy. ATP is reduced to adenosine **di**phosphate (ADP), and one molecule of phosphate floats free. Creatine phosphate immediately leaps in, and regenerates the ATP by donating its own phosphate molecule, leaving a molecule of free creatine in the muscle. The ATP is then able to work again.

After a muscle contraction, most of the free creatine and free phosphate molecules floating around in the muscle join together again to regenerate creatine phosphate. But this process requires oxygen, so you have to stop anaerobic exercise to allow it to happen. After you stop, half the spent creatine is regenerated to creatine phosphate in about 60 seconds. A maximum of 90% is regenerated over a five-minute rest period.[2] The remaining 10% is excreted from the muscles, and appears as the waste product **creatinine** in your urine.

This biochemical scenario is critical for building muscle and strength, because it tells you exactly how long to rest between sets for maximum growth. In order to make the most intense muscle contraction on your next effort, you have to wait until the maximum amount of creatinine has regenerated — about 5 minutes.

Creatine phosphate is the only way to regenerate spent ADP to ATP, and allow near maximum muscle contraction to continue past 4-5 seconds. So you can see immediately the importance of having a full load of creatine phosphate in every muscle.

Creatine Uptake by Muscles

In 1992, Paul Greenhaff of the University of Nottingham, Queen's Medical Center in England, and Roger Harris of the Karolinska Institute in Stockholm, Sweden, and their colleagues, tested the notion that athletes may be short of creatine. They found that a 5- gram oral dose of creatine rapidly raises blood creatine levels. Increasing the dose to 5 grams, 4-6 times daily, they found a big increase in muscle creatine levels.[3]

Studies done over a century ago show that wild animals have much more creatine in their muscles than domesticated animals, a finding attributed to their greater level of exercise.[4] Following these findings, Dr. Harris then made subjects exercise one leg for an hour a day. Creatine level in the exercised leg rose by 50% more than in the unexercised leg.[3]

Recent studies with athletes confirm these findings. Oral creatine supplements increase muscle creatine, and strenuous exercise increases muscle uptake of creatine by about another 50%.[4,5,6] So it's likely that many athletes have sub-optimal levels of creatine in their muscles.

Creatine For Muscle and Strength

The chemistry of creatine tells us just what we might expect from supplementation. For short, intense exercise beyond about 5 seconds, extra muscle creatine should regenerate more ATP, therefore permitting more intense muscle contraction. So as soon as your muscles are loaded with creatine, you should be stronger right away.

Recent research dramatically supports this hypothesis. At Nottingham University in England, Paul Greenhaff and colleagues gave cyclists 4 doses of 5 grams of creatine per day for 5 days and compared them with a placebo. Creatine increased peak power output by 6% during a 30-second maximum effort.[4] That's big!

In another recent study, Conrad Earnest and colleagues at Texas Southwestern Medical Center and The Cooper Clinic in Dallas, gave experienced weight trainers 20 grams of creatine per day for 28 days. They measured performance on the 1-rep maximum bench press. The average increase was 18 lbs, a 6.5 % improvement in strength.[7]

The second prediction from the biochemistry of creatine, is that supplementation will allow you to carry on near maximal exercise for longer, so you should be able to train harder, and therefore generate faster muscle growth.

In the strength study above, Dr. Earnest found that average repetitions at 70% of 1-rep maximum increased from 11 to 15.[7] Paul Balsom and team at the Karolinska Institute also found a significant increase in work output. They tested subjects over 10 sets of 6-second bouts of cycling at two levels of high intensity. Compared with a placebo group, creatine increased the amount of work done at both levels.[8]

This study is a good model of intermittent heavy-weight, low-rep exercise that characterizes the best weight training. By increasing muscle overload the most, it stimulates the greatest adaptive growth. And plenty of growth there was. Over a one-month period Dr. Balsom found increases in lean mass of 0.7 to 5.5 lbs., with an average of 2.4 lbs.[8] Conrad Earnest found even greater growth in his studies. After 28 days of 20 grams of creatine per day, his subjects showed an average increase in lean mass of 3.5 lbs.[7]

In a more recent study , Balsom reports similar increases in mass in *six days* of 20 grams creatine per day.[5] You may see these figures cited in ads, but give them no respect. At the Colgan Institute we have seen similar jumps in bodyweight, only to find later they were mostly water. But 2.4 - 3.5 lbs. over one month is a good bet for real lean tissue growth, and is beyond anything a drug-free athlete can achieve without creatine.

Creatine monohydrate continues to be one of the best supplements for increasing muscle and strength. At the Colgan Institute we have been using the stuff with athletes for the last nine years, and making long-term measurements of results. On average, elite and long experienced athletes, doing four 8-week cycles per year, separated by 4-week rests, show strength gains in their 1-rep maximum squat and dead lift of 15-20% **above** what they were gaining previously without creatine.

If that sounds complicated, here's an example from my files. In 1996 a powerlifter showed a 55-lb gain in his 1-rep max squat without using creatine. After doing creatine during 1997, religiously following the protocol in my creatine book,1 his 1-rep max squat increased by a further 78 lbs. For a man already at the top of his game, that's huge!

Recent studies continue to support these results. Bosco and colleagues at the University of Rome, Italy have just shown that a single-week of creatine monohydrate (20 g daily, 5 days) increased jumping power by 7-12% and sprinting speed by 13%.[10]

It works with women too. Vandenberghe and team at the Katholicke Universiteit in Leuven, Belgium gave healthy young women 20 grams creatine daily for 4 days, or a placebo (20 g daily, 4 days). This short supplement period increased the maximum strength period of the women over a 10-week resistance training program by 20 - 25% more than the placebo.[11]

The latest findings show that creatine also increases ability to perform repeated intermittent maximum efforts. Prevost and colleagues at the Marine Corps Air Station in El Toro gave subjects either 18.75 g creatine monohydrate or a placebo for 5 days, then 2.25 g creatine daily. Then subjects cycled to exhaustion, with the ergometer set for intermittent 10 - sec efforts that would require **150%** of the subject's maximum oxygen uptake. The creatine increased ability to repeat intermittent maximum work by an average of 60% above placebo.12 No wonder it's so good forstrength, because short, intermittent maximum efforts are what strength training is all about.

The latest study is even more exciting, because it applies creatine to longer endurance efforts. Engelhardt and colleagues at Orthopadische Universitatsklinik in Frankfurt, Germany gave experienced triathletes creatine monohydrate (6 g, 5 days). Subjects increased their power in intermittent maximum efforts by 18%.[13]

How Much Creatine?

The daily intake of creatine you need for maximum effect on muscle and strength, depends on how much muscle you have to fill. It also depends on how much exercise you do. I'm assuming that you are training at high intensity, that is 5-days per week or more. If you're not training that hard, then increasing your training will have more effect than creatine or any other ergogenic supplement, so don't waste your money. Studies show that resistance exercise for an hour a day raises muscle creatine the most.[3] To get the benefits from creatine you have to train – hard.

Some guides to creatine use, use bodyweight to calculate creatine need.[9] It's a poor measure because folk vary widely in bodyfat. Bodyfat doesn't need creatine. Over 95% of body creatine is in your muscles. At the Colgan Institute we use muscle weight as the major criterion. Muscle weight in athletes is about 50% of lean weight in men and 35% of lean weight in women. So, in order to find out your personal creatine requirement, you have to know your **lean weight**, that is, your bodyweight minus your fat weight.

Studies in the early '90s found that low doses of creatine didn't raise muscle creatine much.[3] We have found the same results for blood creatine levels in single case studies. So there's some justification for loading creatine at the beginning of a cycle. Whether this strategy is essential to trigger super-loading of the muscles, is still being investigated. Until the evidence is out, loading is in.

We use a 6-day creatine loading regimen, with 0.5 grams of creatine per kilogram **muscle** weight. To save you the sums, the daily amount of creatine for loading, based on your **lean** weight, and high intensity training, is given in the table below.

Table 6:
Creatine Loading and Maintenance

Lean Bodyweight		Males		Females	
lbs	kg	Loading gms	Maintenance gms	Loading gms	Maintenance gms
80	36	9	3	6	2
100	45	11	3.5	8	2.5
120	55	14	4.5	10	3
140	64	16	5	11.5	3.5
160	73	18	6	13	4
180	82	20	6.5	14.5	4.5
200	91	22.5	7	16	5
220	100	25	8	17.5	6

Sources: Colgan Institute, San Diego, 1996

Once you are loaded, it doesn't take a lot of creatine to keep you there. There's some evidence from Paul Balsom that subjects at unspecified levels of exercise, need only 10% of the loading dose.[6] In case studies of athletes exercising at high intensity, we have found this amount insufficient. Until better controlled evidence comes out, we have adopted 25% of the loading dose as the maintenance criterion. Maintenance doses are also given in the table. That's all the creatine you'll ever need.

Divided Doses

The best way to load creatine is, divided doses, taken at spaced intervals throughout the day. Divide your daily intake into four. Take one dose 30-60 minutes before workout. Creatine is then digested and in the bloodstream by the time you begin exercise.

Take anther dose immediately after workout. After exercise your muscles are hungry for creatine. so if you get into the bloodstream within 30 minutes after workout, you get a further edge in muscle uptake. Take the other two doses spaced out to fill the day.

Sugar Is Essential

The second strategy is sugar. You enhance muscle uptake of creatine by taking each dose with an 8 oz drink containing 30 - 40 grams of mixed sugars. The sugars stimulate the insulin that is essential to push creatine through muscle cell membranes.

We use a 50:50 mix of grape juice and grapefruit juice. Grapefruit juice contains acids and enzymes that reduce stomach acidity by stimulating the pancreas to release acid buffering chemicals.

Boost Insulin Efficiency

The third strategy is to maximize insulin efficiency. In almost all the research and in some case studies at the Colgan Institute, some individuals showed increased blood creatine levels, but no increase in muscle or strength. Various researchers suggest this failure may be caused by inefficient insulin metabolism,[9] or insulin resistance,[7] whereby insulin fails in its normal task of moving chemicals through the cell membrane.

When we examined the nutrition and blood profiles of our non-responders, we found two prominent problems. First, most of their diets contained insufficient chromium for normal insulin metabolism. Many of them also showed somewhat elevated blood sugar, blood insulin, and blood triglycerides, the classic symptom trilogy of insulin resistance. When we add the known insulin potentiators, 400-800 mcg of chromium picolinate, 300-600 mg of omega-3 fatty acids, and 100 mg of alpha-lipoic acid to the creatine mix, many of our failures become successes.

We also use 25 mg of dehydroepiandrosterone (DHEA). Levels of this hormone begin to decline after age 20, and recent research shows that supplementation with 25 mg per day, restores youthful levels and enhances insulin efficiency.[14]

Cycle Creatine

Finally, you should cycle creatine. No one knows whether continuous creatine supplementation interferes with the body's own ability to make creatine, or whether the human body adapts to the supplements over long-term use, so that muscle creatine declines to its former level. Until that research is done, we cycle creatine over 8 weeks with a 4-week rest.

As with all supplements that have big effects on body function, where evidence of long-term safety is lacking, we treat the chemical with respect. You should too. If you follow this article to help you use creatine, you should first read the scientific references. Even then, you use it at your own choice and risk.

What Form of Creatine?

With such reliable results extending to every kind of athlete and sport, it's no wonder that companies selling creatine will do anything to increase their market share. Various kinds of creatine, especially creatine citrate and creatine pyruvate, compete with creatine mixed with everything from ginseng and royal jelly to adenosine triphosphate. Then there's liquid creatine, super stable creatine, creatine serum, creatine chews, creatine tablets, Old Uncle Tom Cobbly and All.

Latest to hit the market is effervescent creatine. This product provides a telling example of what happens in the sports supplement industry, as companies try to gain a commercial edge, with little thought for efficacy of the product, and with no thought at all for the athletes who buy it. So I want to spell it out in detail to help you avoid being fooled by the many bogus claims we see all the time in product advertisements.

Effervescent creatine sounds exotic but it is simply creatine mono-hydrate mixed with plain old bicarbonate of soda and citric acid. As with various effervescent salts on the medical market, it's sup-posed to increase creatine absorption. Give me a break! Creatine monohydrate is well absorbed anyway without fizzing it.

Back in 1992, Paul Greenhaff at the University of Nottingham in England and Roger Harris of the Karolinska Institute in Stockholm, Sweden clearly showed that a single dose of 5 grams of creatine monohydrate rapidly raises blood and muscle levels of creatine.[3] Feeding athletes six doses of 5 grams per day, they found that 40% of the creatine was excreted on Day 1 rising to 68% by Day 3.[6] Their data show that the human body absorbs creatine so well that it satu-rates in less than a week. Absorption of creatine is not a problem to worry about.

Advertisers of effervescent creatine also make big play about non-responders, claiming that their creatine will solve the problem. After nine years of studying creatine, I can tell you it's not the absorption or the form of creatine that causes some athletes to fail to respond. The most common problem we and other researchers have found with non-responders to creatine is insulin resistance, or inefficient insulin metabolism.[7,9]

The last-ditch play in ads for effervescent creatine is a "clinical study performed at a leading university," purporting to show that their creatine caused a 28.9% increase in "anaerobic working capacity," compared with a 15.7% increase for creatine monohydrate with carbs."

Just to be sure I was not missing the boat, I got my staff to search all journals on the Internet and to contact all the leading creatine researchers. Here's a condensed version of what a couple of the top researchers had to say in reply to our query. First, is the original guy who discovered creatine's benefits for sports, Dr. Paul Greenhaff of Nottingham University Medical School, Nottingham, England.

"I have no information about this product. I can see no reason why it would be any more effective at increasing muscle creatine retention than powder form creatine dissolved in water."

Paul Greenhaff
24 December 1998.

Another top researcher is Dr. Richard Kreider of the University of Memphis, Tennessee.

"I am not aware of any study which has compared the effectiveness of effervescent creatine to creatine monohydrate on muscle uptake. Intestinal absorption of creatine is not a limiting factor. Once absorbed, the muscle then takes up what is needed to top off muscle levels. Once loaded, extra creatine is eliminated primarily through urinary excretion. Unless I see data to show that muscle creatine content is increased to a greater degree with effervescent creatine, I would be skeptical of these claims."

Richard Kreider
29 December 1998.

Following these reports, the continuing efforts of my staff to track down data brought an e-mail response from Dr Jeffrey Stout of Creighton University in Omaha, NE. Dr. Stout and team had done one **pilot** study comparing effervescent creatine monohydrate with powder creatine monohydrate. This study was unpublished but is the one cited in effervescent creatine advertisements. To show you that I am not hedging or changing anything, here are Dr Stout's own words regarding effervescent creatine.

"As you know creatine supplementation appears to have non-responders as well as responders on performance measures. So far we have seen 100% success with Eff-cr as compared 70% success with powder. This would explain why the mean values for the Eff-cr were so much larger. However, if you compare only the success values between the powder creatine and eff-cr there was no significant difference between them."[15]

As you can see, straight from the horse's mouth, effervescent creatine did not achieve greater growth of muscle and strength. The success claimed in ads for effervescent creatine, is simply an artifact of having no non responders in the effervescent creatine group. Without the non-responders who lowered the average success of the powder creatine group by scoring 0, the **average** success of the effervescent creatine group is, of course higher. Dr. Stout probably did the further analysis showing no difference in degree of success between groups because he also saw this obvious artifact. *Caveat Emptor*

There's not a scrap of scientific evidence that any other creatine works better than plain creatine monohydrate taken with appropriate carbs. In fact, with all the other compounds arbitrarily mixed with creatine in some of these products, it's likely they don't work as well. Almost all the studies to date have been done with creatine monohydrate, which is therefore the sole and only form of creatine for which we have scientific evidence of effectiveness.

There is a lot of bad creatine out there, and, if you've been having problems, it's probably the bargain brand you're using. All the good brands are very fine powder, with virtually no taste, no grit, no smell, and no side-effects.

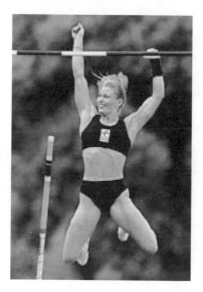

Emma George, world champion in the pole vault 15 feet off the ground – flying by human power and loving it.

45

GLUCOSAMINE AND CHONDROITIN

In Volume 2 of this series I cover the use of essential fats for soft tissue injuries. Here I want to cover three other important components, glucosamine sulfate, chondroitin sulfate, and S-adenosylmethionine. Together with essential fats, they are a real breakthrough for those sore shoulders, elbows, hips, backs, knees and ankles. Once you feel the benefits, you won't leave home without them.

The Glucosamine Limit

Cartilage, the tough, spongy cushion between the ends of your bones and some other soft tissues, are mostly composed of collagen fibrils and feathery strings called **proteoglycans**. These are replaced continuously in response to the wear and tear of exercise. The rate-limiting chemical step in proteoglycans production is **glucosamine**. Thus, together with collagen, glucosamine determines how quickly your joints can repair themselves and recover from the stress of intense weight-bearing stress.

Your body makes glucosamine from glucose and the amino acid glutamine. Glutamine, produced mainly in your muscles, or eaten in food, is in constant demand by your muscles, your immune system and your joints. Athletes are hard put to get enough of it. My book *Optimum Sports Nutrition* documents how intense exercise can easily overwhelm your glutamine supply.[1] Joints are often left short, so that strains, pains, synovitis, bursitis, and all sorts of other "itises" are quick to develop and slow to heal.

You can bypass the joint shortage by taking glucosamine sulfate supplements, thereby providing glucosamine ready-made for production of proteoglycans. Animal studies show that oral glucosamine can increase proteoglycans by up to 170%.[2,3] This increase has big benefits for aching joints. I can cover only a smidgen of the studies in this short chapter, but will do my best to provide examples that represent the overall evidence.

Most of the research has been on patients diagnosed with osteoarthritis. A typical study was done on arthritic knees by Dr. Antonio Vaz at St. Johns Hospital in Oporto, Portugal. In a double-blind trial, he gave subjects either 1.5 grams daily of glucosamine sulfate or 1.2 grams of the non-steroidal anti-inflammatory drug ibuprofen (Advil). The glucosamine group showed greater relief of pain and better recovery of function than the ibuprofen group.[4]

In a representative study of athletes, 51 males and 17 females with cartilage damage of the knees were given 1500 mg of glucosamine sulfate daily for 40 days, then 750 mg daily for another 100 days. Of the 68 athletes, 52 showed complete cure of their injury and resumed full training. A follow-up 12 months later showed no sign of cartilage damage in any of them.[5]

Glucosamine came to my rescue too, for a left knee injury sustained while deadlifting a new personal record. The MRI showed both cartilages torn, the anterior cruciate ligament torn half through and the lateral colateral ligament hanging on by a thread. Medical diagnosis: no chance of a functional knee again without surgery. I refused the surgery, because the evidence shows that it leads almost inevitably to arthritis later in life. Instead, I used a ton of glucosamine, 10 grams or more a day, plus essential fats and mega-antioxidants to bowel tolerance. With a lot of special rehab weight work using the Power Program, the knee healed over four months and returned to full function in just under a year. Now, eight years later, I have no problems with it, neither when lifting nor when running.

The Chondroitin Dilemma

Chondroitin is another important biochemical manufactured in your joints. In conjunction with sulfur, it forms a big part of the protoglycans structure of cartilage. It acts also to assist synovial fluid to lubricate the cartilage.

Chondroitin and synovial fluid both decline in numerous arthritic disorders. The cartilage loses bulk and progressively dries out, becoming stiff and scratchy like a kitchen scouring pad.[6] The sliding surfaces eventually become like sandpaper, especially if crystals of uric acid, calcium pyrophosphate or other minerals have infiltrated the joint. So it is a reasonable idea to try to overcome these problems with supplements of chondroitin sulfate.

Trouble is, chondroitin sulfate has a hard job getting through your intestinal wall and into the bloodstream. With a molecular weight of about 30,000 for most preparations of the compound, the chondroitin molecule is far too big. In contrast, glucosamine sulfate has a molecular weight of just 211, and passes through the wall like ants up a trouser leg.

Nevertheless, animal studies in the 1980's, using radioactively-labeled chondroitin, showed increased levels of radioactivity in the blood, suggesting that it was somehow getting through.[7,8] This work led to wild claims for chondroitin as the answer to arthritis, and it's distribution worldwide as a nutritional supplement. More sophisticated recent work, however, on rabbits and on human subjects, shows negligible absorption of intact chondroitin.[6,9,10]

Nevertheless, studies with rats and men, using oral doses of radioactively-labeled chondroitin, continue to show increases in the blood of chondroitin-related and proteoglycan-related molecules.[11] Many of these molecules, however, are still too big to have passed in from the gut. Most likely they are reconstructed in the blood from small molecular components which are released from chondroitin when it is broken down by digestion. One of these small components is glucosamine sulfate. Your body performs this construction miracle continually with many of the nutrients you eat every day.

Research with new, more sensitive methods of analysis support the idea that the body does it for chondroitin. In a representative study, Dr L Silvestro and colleagues at Res Pharma in Torino, Italy, examined the changes in blood proteoglycans after oral doses of chondroitin sulfate in healthy men. They showed that numerous proteoglycans-like substances appeared in the blood. They also showed that some of them had totally lost their sulfur content, indicating they had been broken down, most likely in the gut, and then reconstructed without sulfur in the blood.[12]

More Chondroitin Benefits

Other recent studies show two more beneficial effects of oral chondroitin sulfate. It can raise blood levels of another important compound called **hyaluronan**[13], which, in your joints, is a sticky gel that cements the tissues together. Chondroitin can also increase collagen formation in joints. Remember, we saw earlier that collagen fibrils and proteoglycans together form the structure of cartilage.[13,14]

So, although I have been skeptical of chondroitin in earlier writings, and have thought that its reliable, though moderate benefits[15] were a result of the glucosamine it released, I have to bow to the science. Although it may not be absorbed intact, there are benefits of chondroitin for arthritis in addition to those conferred by glucosamine.

S-adenosylmethionine Breakthrough

Few folk yet know about **S-adenosylmethionine** (SAMe), yet to biochemists it ranks almost equal in importance with the primary energy molecule adenosine triphosphate (ATP). SAMe works in almost every cell as the active form in which your body uses the essential amino acid methionine. It performs such a wide variety of functions it would take a book to describe them. Here we are concerned only with its benefit for joint problems. It's a biggie.

Using glucosamine in conjunction with essential fats over the last decade, we have had a success rate with arthritis patients and with athletes of about 60%. In 1994, when nutrition advocates finally pushed through the Hatch Act, which allows all Americans free access to nutrient supplements, many previously banned substances became available, including SAMe. Since then we have added SAMe to all our treatment protocols for injuries and inflammatory conditions of the joints, with a big increase in success.

Initial studies with animals showed conclusively that intra-muscular injections of SAMe increased the number of chondrocytes in cartilage, and the thickness of the cartilage pad.[16] Remember, the chondrocyte is the only living element in cartilage. It produces all the proteoglycans and collagen that make up the cartilage structure. So any nutrient that can increase the number of chondrocytes should be seized upon with glee. The big question was, does it work orally?

The answer came in more animal studies in the mid '80s which demonstrated easy intestinal absorption of oral SAMe, and subsequent anti-inflammatory and analgesic actions.[17] Armed with this evidence researchers throughout the world set to work.

Extensive studies in Italy with 22,000 arthritis patients over five years showed unequivocally that SAMe increases proteoglycans production by chondrocytes in human cartilage, with no toxicity and virtually no side-effects.[18] Most of these studies are with patients classified as osteoarthritic. But SAMe also has beneficial effects for rheumatoid conditions. One of the classic signs of rheumatoid problems is an auto-immune attack on the joint and synovial membrane, especially by the potent immune component tumor necrosis factor (TNF). In 1997 researchers in Spain published important results in the British Journal of Rheumatology, showing that SAMe restores synovial cells after they are damaged by TNF. It's specific effects on TNF action suggest that using SAMe to prevent synovial damage may be an even better way to go.[19]

SAMe Beats NSAIDs

Another great advantage of SAMe is that it reduces pain and loss of function sufficiently to enable patients to stop using the usual NSAIDs. As I've discussed elsewhere NSAIDs may reduce pain but they also inhibit healing.[20] Thus SAMe helps enormously to set up the ideal conditions for joints to repair themselves. Here are a couple of examples of the evidence.

In a double-blind comparison at the famous Arthritis Clinic in Bad Abbach in Germany, patients diagnosed with arthritic conditions of the knees, hips, and spine, were given either 1200 mg of SAMe or 1200 mg of ibuprofen daily for four weeks. Clinical results of the two treatments were equal for reduction of pain, swelling and stiffness, and for increase in range of motion.[21]

A similar double-blind clinical trial compared 1200 mg of SAMe with the tolerable dose of 750 mg of naproxsyn (Naprosyn). Both treatments had equal effects on pain, but SAMe caused fewer side-effects and was judged the better treatment all round.[22]

SAMe Aids Joint Regeneration

Another important finding came from research on arthritis of the knee by Dr. A. Maccagno at Hospital Frances in Buenos Aires, Argentina. He showed not only that SAMe produced equal clinical results to the drug piroxicam, but also that patients given SAMe maintained the improvements in symptoms and in function for a considerable period after SAMe was withdrawn. Improvements quickly faded after piroxicam was withdrawn. This continuation of function after SAMe is further supporting evidence that the nutrient is helping to rebuild the joint.[23]

The longest controlled study with SAMe continued for two years. Under the control of Dr. B. Konig at the University of Maintz in Germany, 10 physicians in various parts of Germany treated 108 patients diagnosed with chronic arthritis of knees, hips, and spine. Patients received 600 mg of SAMe daily for 4 weeks, then only 400 mg per day for the rest of two years. Even with this small dosage, clinical improvements began within about one week and continued, in many cases progressively, for the whole two-year period. Examinations at 6, 12, 18 and 24 months showed no further arthritic degeneration, indicating that SAMe was assisting joint repair and was preventing progress of the disease. More important, 18 patients with long-term arthritic problems showed total remission of symptoms.[24]

There are no controlled studies yet of S-adenosylmethionine with athletes. But our experience of adding it to our joint regimen, plus the research evidence, examples of which are reviewed above, is sufficient to convince me of its efficacy against all sorts of soft tissue damage and inflammation. A typical day's supplementation for stubborn knee, shoulder, elbow, and hip and back problems is shown below. The regimen takes a while to show benefits, but persistence for twelve weeks, plus the right rehab exercise, often brings complete remission.

Typical Colgan Institute Joint Regimen

On rising in A.M.   2-4 tablespoons organic flax oil in
                       protein shake

With Breakfast   2 capsules (1000 mg size)
                          gamma linolenic acid
                       2 capsules (1000 mg size)
                          eicosapentaenoic acid
                       1000 mg glucosamine sulfate
                       200 mg S-adenosylmethionine
                       500 mg chondroitin sulfate

With Lunch   3 capsules gamma linolenic acid
                       3 capsules eicosapentaenoic acid
                       1000 mg glucosamine sulfate
                       200 mg S-adenosylmethionine
                       500 mg chondroitin sulfate

With Dinner   3 capsules gamma linolenic acid
                       3 capsules eicosapentaenoic acid
                       1000 mg glucasmine sulfate
                       200 mg S-adenosylmethionine
                       500 mg chondroitin sulfate

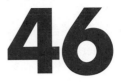

SOY ISOFLAVONES

Japanese women have small breasts. Japanese men have small prostates. Compared to Americans that is, even Americans of Japanese descent. Japanese also enjoy much lower rates of breast and prostate cancer. Unless they migrate to America that is, where their rates for those cancers rise rapidly towards the whopping US levels.[1,2]

Discovery of these anomalies in the '60s, led scientists to search for dietary differences between Japanese and Americans, that might be causing certain cancers in America and protecting folk against them in Japan. The data base grew quickly to include colon cancer, endometrial cancer, high cholesterol, heart disease, osteoporosis, menopause and adult-onset diabetes. All the evidence was in in Japan's favor.[1] Despite their overcrowding and high levels of environmental pollution, low rates of these diseases have now made the Japanese the longest-lived people on Earth. They have an average lifespan of 80 years, longer than any Scandinavian country, and *four years* longer than Americans.[3]

No, it's not a genetic difference between races, because second generation Japanese-Americans suffer roughly the same disease rates as other Americans, and live no longer than the American average. To cut a long story short, the only difference that crops up constantly to explain Japan's superior health, is the preponderance of vegetable protein in their diets.

The Trouble With Meat

Americans get a surfeit of chicken soup for the soul, but it's not doing our bodies a whole lot of good. Our high animal protein diets, with the highest rates of chicken and beef consumption in the world, are crucifying our health. Let's take the example of cardiovascular disease. Over 96,000,000 adult Americans, that's more than half the total adult population, now have blood cholesterol levels over 200 mg/dl (5.2 mmol/l). Nearly 38,000,000 have levels over 240 mg/dl (6.2 mmol/l).[4] Just to remind you, risk of cardiovascular disease starts to rise at a cholesterol level of 168 mg/dl (4.4 mmol/l). At 240 mg/dl, you are a walking time-bomb for a heart attack.[3] The average American Joe is one sick puppy.

"So what?" you say. "I'm healthy, low bodyfat, train regularly, fit as a flea. I'm not your average Joe." No you're not an average Joe. Athletes need even **more** animal protein than average Joes. And even though you peel every scrap of skin off your chicken breasts, that extra protein whacks you good. We took a sample off the Colgan Institute computer record of the cholesterol levels of 100 drug-free athletes we have worked with. Average cholesterol was 204 mg/dl (5.3 mmol/l), well into the range of cardiovascular risk.

How can this be, when we all eat a low-fat, low-cholesterol diet and exercise enough to bust a gut? Athletes are closer to the US health authorities advice for heart health than any other group in the nation. Sorry folk but I have to explode another health myth. Medical thinking and public belief, are still stuck on the notion that high levels of fats in food, especially saturated animal fats and ***trans***-fats, are the only causes of high cholesterol worth worrying about. It's all a load of 30-years-out-of-date cobblers.

True, a high-fat diet will send your cholesterol over the moon. But its not just the fat that does it. The fat may not even be the main cause. The National Cholesterol Education Program Diet, which embodies low-fat, low-cholesterol food, achieves only a modest 10% reduction in high cholesterol levels.[5] I have to tell you that recent evidence shows that the animal protein itself disorders cholesterol metabolism.[6-8]

Those Pesky Hormones

I only have space to give you a taste of the reasons why animal proteins increase cholesterol levels. A big one, that all athletes should know, is that the amino acid structure of the proteins you eat has potent effects on your hormones. Most athletes are familiar with using single amino acids such as L-arginine and ornithine alpha-ketoglutarate to increase growth hormone output. But few that I ask, have made the connection between these effects and the amino acids in intact proteins. Knowing just what aminos do, can not only help your heart, but can also save you a lot of grief in the gym.

All the usual meats we eat contain high levels of the amino acid L-lysine but only moderate levels of L-arginine. L-lysine strongly opposes the growth-hormone releasing, muscle-building, fat-reducing effects of L-arginine. In fact L-lysine acts on your hormones much like a high-fat diet. It increases insulin production and reduces glucagon production by the pancreas. This change in the ratio in insulin to glucagon, signals your liver to make fat and cholesterol like crazy.[9,10]   If you add L-lysine to animal diets, their cholesterol levels increase by over 50%, and they plump up like Pooh Bear.[9,10]

Now you know why smart guys in sports medicine, advocate additional L-arginine or OKG with every animal protein meal. If you've been doing everything else right but just can't shift that body-fat, or get your cholesterol down to 150, L-lysine in your meat is one likely culprit.

Soy To The Rescue

As I've documented numerous times, soy protein isolate has a lower biological value (BV) than whey proteinisolate. It doesn't generate near as much muscle as the recently developed whey peptides.[11] But soy has other advantages which makes it a valuable food for athletes. First, soy protein contains a lower lysine to arginine ratio than meats. Numerous recent studies show that substitution of 30 grams of soy protein daily for a meat meal, reduces the insulin to glucagon ratio, increases blood levels of arginine, and dramatically reduces cholesterol levels.[2] Now you might start to realize why the soy-eating Japanese outlive us.

There are no studies on athletes yet to confirm bodyfat reduction by soy. But most of the fat-reducing claims of the popular Zone Diet for endurance athletes, hinge on reducing the insulin to glucagon ratio. The Zone Diet is complicated and too high in fat for most athletes. Soy is simple and may do the job in a snip.

Isoflavones For Breast Health

Soy also contains the isoflavones **genestein** and **diadzein**, which offer potent protection for athletes against a variety of ills. Here's a sampling of the latest studies, presented at the recent International Medical Conference on Soy, held in Brussels, Belgium.[2] I will group them in order of the physical characteristics and health advantages of Japanese citizens, noted at the start of this article.

First is breast size and breast cancer. Studies of human breast cells by Dr. Stephen Barnes and colleagues at the University of Alabama, show that genestein from soy strongly inhibits breast growth in healthy breast tissue.[2] More important, genestein also prevents proliferation of many types of human breast cancer cells. Dr. Dolores Foth and colleagues at Universitat Griefswald, in Germany, report similar findings in female macaque monkeys fed isoflavone-enriched soy protein isolate. In addition, they found that the soy inhibited both breast and endometrial growth.[2]

An extensive epidemiological study supports these findings. Dr. Anna Wu and colleagues at the University of Southern California in Los Angeles, studied breast cancer rates of Chinese-American, Japanese-American, and Filipino-American women in Los Angeles and Hawaii. They found that the higher the tofu intake, the lower the breast cancer rate. These and similar findings reported at the Brussels conference[2], indicate that soy isoflavones may be the major variable in the smaller breast size and much lower breast cancer rates of Japanese women.

I always thought that the Western idolatry of massive mammaries, was one of the silliest excursions of man's tendency to vulgarize female anatomy. Breast cancer is the most frequent form of cancer in American women. Big boobs also inhibit athletic performance, by their weight, their wind resistance, and their tendency to flop around. Female athletes can gain a performance edge by adding tofu, miso and soy protein isolate to their nutrition, with the added bonus of potent protection against breast cancer.

Prostate Protection

Male athletes are always trying to increase testosterone levels. And their levels are a lot higher than the average. By itself, weight training increases testosterone levels. And so does muscle mass. For muscle and strength it's a dandy idea. For health it's risky business.

Anything that increases testosterone, increases the risk of high dihydrotestosterone levels and stimulation of prostate growth. Overgrowth of your prostate doesn't always lead to cancer, but I wouldn't bet on it. Cancer aside, I've seen too many 40-year-old-plus athletes, driven crazy by prostatitis and other prostate problems. Regular use of soy may be all that they need.

Researchers at the Department of Urology at South Manchester University Hospital in England, fed normal prostate cells and prostate cancer cells genestein and diadzein. The soy isoflavones inhibited normal prostate cell growth and ***completely stopped*** the cancer cell growth. Soy is likely a major reason why most Japanese men keep their prostates small and untrammeled for life.

Soy For Bones

Athletes train to extremes these days in order to feature among the elite. This training reduces estrogen in women and testosterone in men, and also induces mineral deficiencies. These changes are sufficient to cause rapid bone loss in both males and females, and are a major factor in the high rate of stress fractures in athletes.

As discussed in the chapters on minerals, this bone loss can be inhibited by mineral supplementation. But there's no doubt that hormones are also involved. Anabolic hormone manipulation, however, is neither desirable nor permissible for drug-free athletes. Soy may provide an effective alternative.

Multiple animal and human studies presented at the Brussels conference, show that genestein from soy prevents bone loss[2]. Dr. Harry Blair at the University of Alabama, for example, reported that genestein specifically reduces formation of **osteoclasts**, the cells that degrade bone. Dr. John Anderson and team at the University of North Carolina, showed that genestein saves as much bone as an equivalent dose of estradiol (estrogen), and with none of estrogen's toxic effects. Dr. John Erdman at the University of Illinois, showed that 40 grams a day of soy isolate protein, containing 90 mg total isoflavones, significantly increased bone density in post-menopausal women. Soy seems smart thinking as a supplement for bones.

Soy Is Antioxidant

Soy isoflavones have a long reach. They influence many systems throughout the body. One way that genestein inhibits cardiovascular disease for example, is by inhibiting platelet aggregation and the oxidation of low-density lipoproteins, the starting phases of atherosclerosis. Dr. Norberta Schone from the USDA Human Nutrition Center in Beltsville, Maryland, reports that genestein neutralizes free radicals in blood platelets. Dr. Takemishi Kanazawa of Hirosaki School of Medicine, Japan, reports that soy strongly inhibits LDL oxidation. With the enormous free radical load produced by exercise, athletes need all the food-borne antioxidants they can get.

Soy Is Diuretic

Athletes are forever asking the Colgan Institute how to lose water to make weight just prior to contests, without using dangerous diuretics or getting the weakness that comes from sweating it out in the sauna. I covered various ways of doing it in *Optimum Sports Nutrition*.[12] One thing I didn't cover is soy.

Interesting new evidence comes from RM Martinez and colleagues at the Zaragosa Faculty of Medicine in Spain. Following previous reports that soy isoflavones improve kidney function in diabetes and other disorders, they compared genestein with the strong loop diuretic drug **furosemide**. In rat kidney tissue, the isoflavone produced a diuretic effect equal to that of the drug[2]. No studies exist in healthy humans yet, but it looks promising.

Gender Differences

From its effects on female breast and endometrial tissue, you may have guessed by now, that the isoflavone genestein belongs to that class of chemicals loosely called **phytoestrogens**. This gobbledegook term simply means chemicals from plants with estrogenic activity in animals. This activity has prompted some writers to warn male athletes against soy isoflavones, claiming they are estrogen mimics that will distort hormone balance and whack hard-earned muscle. They are dead wrong.

In a representative study, Dr. L J Lul and team at the University of Texas in Galveston, gave men and pre-menopausal women 1000 mg genestein and 100 mg diadzein daily for a month, contained in soy milk. They measured their hormones up, down, and sideways. In these women, estrogen levels dropped by 60%, and progesterone levels dropped by 35%. These hormone changes support the beneficial effects of soy isoflavones in preventing overgrowth of breast tissue and preventing breast and endometrial cancer.

In men, however, both estrogen and testosterone levels remained unchanged; but metabolites of dihydrotestosterone, which promotes prostate overgrowth, declined by 13%. Other markers of possible pre-cancerous changes in the prostate declined by up to 60 %.

These and similar findings in other studies prompt two conclusions. First, they support the evidence that soy isoflavones inhibit the conversion of testosterone to dihydrotestosterone, and thus reduce prostate overgrowth, and reduce the risk of prostate cancer. Second, they indicate clear gender differences in the action of these isoflavones.

Animal studies confirm these gender differences. Normal male rats injected with diadzcin, show big rises in growth hormone and testosterone levels and increased muscle gain. Normal female rats show big declines in growth hormone and testosterone levels and reduced muscle gain.[13] Soy isoflavones don't appear to have any detectable estrogenic action in males, action that would be detrimental to anabolic hormones or muscle.

Use The Right Soy

Soy products differ enormously in their isoflavone content. Some soy proteins are cheaply produced by alcohol extraction from the beans. This process removes most of the isoflavones. Modern mass-produced, low-fat versions of traditional soy foods such as tofu, also lose more than half their isoflavones in processing.[14] Many soy products that try to imitate Western foods, such as bacon, sausages, and burgers have been rooted, tooted, roasted, toasted, and chemically lambasted until there's nothing left.

In contrast, traditional Japanese fermented soy foods not only retain their isoflavones, but render them more bioavailable.[15] Good water-extracted soy protein isolate also retains its essential nature.[13] These are the right stuff.

You don't have to eat a lot. Traditional oriental soy products or soy protein isolate, yielding 30 grams of soy protein a day, provides everything you need for the isoflavone advantage.[2]

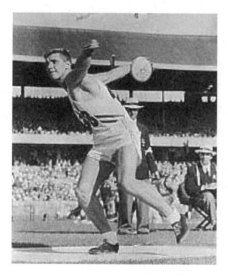

Al Oerter, seen here winning his first Olympic gold medal in the discus in 1956, is the finest example of the persistence to which athletes should aspire. He won the gold in four successive Olympics.

PYGEUM, SAW PALMETTO

A normal prostate gland is about the size and shape of a walnut, dangling below your bladder and wrapped around your urinary tract (urethra). Trouble is, not many of us have normal prostates. More than half of all American males over forty have enlarged prostates.[1] This degenerative condition, called benign prostatic hypertrophy (BPH), squeezes the bladder and urethra makes the victim highly susceptible to urinary tract and bladder infections.

As it progresses, urinary pain, urinary urgency, frequent urination at night, painful sexual activity, reduced sexual potency, and prostatitis force sufferers into a vicious cycle of symptomatic relief by antibiotics and other treatments such as finasteride (Proscar®). Meanwhile, the disorder progresses inexorably and greatly increases the risk of prostate cancer.[2]

"What's that got to do with me?" you say. "I'm a young, healthy bodybuilder." I have to tell you that bodybuilders and athletes in general form a special class that suffers from BPH earlier in life and more severely than Mr. American average. Why? Because athletes, especially strength athletes, have higher levels of testosterone than average Joes, and also take all sorts of chemicals to further boost testosterone.

Testosterone is the main villain in BPH. The prostate contains high levels of an enzyme, **5-alpha-reductase**, which converts testosterone to **dihydrotestosterone (DHT)**. The higher your testosterone level the more DHT the prostate manufactures. DHT grows the prostate like Topsy.[3]

At the Colgan Institute we have seen numerous cases of athletes in their 20s and early 30s, with prostates the size of oranges and symptoms to suit. Most of these guys had been actively boosting testosterone, and irritating the bejesus out of their prostates. Some used testosterone itself or other steroids, some used stimulant herbals falsely claimed to be anabolic, such as yohimbine, others simply worked out hard with weights. From close questioning of a large number of subjects over the last decade, we conclude that symptoms of beginning BPH are common in young athletes.

The only way to prevent degenerative conditions is to catch them early. That's why I put the supplement pygeum/saw palmetto in the "must have" category for male athletes. Before telling you how it works, I want to make an important point about herbals in general, because if you don't know it, you may find yourself stripped of the right to buy them freely and cheap.

The pharmaceutical industry has embarked on a clever campaign to bring certain effective herbals under their profit umbrella of prescription drugs. A big part of this campaign, is to convince the public that these herbals are at best marginal and at worst toxic, and should therefore be closely regulated. The campaign involves many millions of dollars in grants and other perks to medical schools and physicians to write appropriate public pieces. So you may have read in the popular press, or in those non-peer reviewed medical school newsletters, which have proliferated recently as part of drug industry ploys, that pygeum/saw palmetto is "unproven."

Having no advertisers to satisfy, nor profits to pursue, and accepting no grants from drug companies, I am free to tell you the truth. The truth is, pygeum and saw palmetto are both well proven to prevent and even to reverse benign prostatic hypertrophy. Pygeum (Pygeum africanum), the powdered bark of an evergreen African tree, has been used for many centuries to treat urinary problems. Forty years ago European scientists developed an extract containing three groups of chemicals, that reduce prostate inflammation, and edema (swelling), and reduce testosterone uptake by the prostate.[4,5]

Saw palmetto is an extract from the berries of two varieties of fan palm, Sabal serrulata and Serenoa repens, that grow wild across the Southern United States, and in parts of Europe. European scientists established in the '60s, that saw palmetto reduces levels of DHT in the prostate, mainly by inhibiting the enzyme 5-alpha-reductase.[6,7]

Pygeum and saw palmetto, either alone or in combination, have been an approved treatment for BPH in Europe since 1970. A pile of clinical studies in peer-reviewed mainstream journals, show them to be effective in increasing urinary flow, reducing prostate size, reducing prostate inflammation, relieving prostatitis, reducing night-time urination and relieving urinary and sexual pain.[4-9]

For those suffering BPH already, we recommend an extract containing 200 mg of pygeum standardized to 13% total sterols, plus 200 mg of saw palmetto oil, twice daily with food. For athletes without BPH, or with only minor symptoms, the same extract once daily is plenty. Because dihydrotestosterone is also a potent cause of male pattern baldness, this supplement could also save your hair. We have used pygeum/saw palmetto with more than 500 athletes over the past 12 years with very favorable feedback.

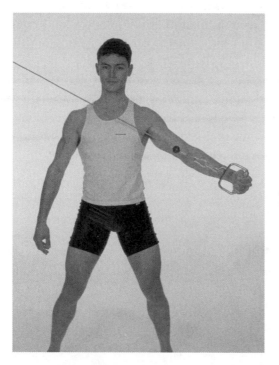

Top trainer Steven Macramalla demonstrating a rotator cuff exercise from the Colgan Power Program.

48

SAVE YOUR BREATH

You eat the best low-fat, low-glycemic, high-protein organically grown food. You never take man-made drugs. You drink and cook with purified water. You take complete vitamins and minerals every day. You balance your strength workouts with aerobics, running, cycling, swimming, or jiggling up and down in the gym on a wondrous assortment of shiny machines. It's the new American myth of the healthy, athletic urban lifestyle. By neglecting the source of one basic component of life - oxygen, you will never reach your potential.

Without oxygen from the environment, you would die within minutes. But in order to get this vital gas today, most of us also have to breathe carbon monoxide, sulfur dioxide, nitrogen oxides, and a smoldering waste dump of poisonous man-made gases. All those joggers I see, running down the grass median strip of Santa Monica Boulevard in their morning pursuit of health, are doing their bodies a lot more harm than good. With the exertion of running, they are breathing 12-20 times the air of sedentary folk. There is no way the benefits of nutrition and exercise can overcome the damage caused by sucking in that much chemical soup. They'd be better off spending an extra hour in bed.

I arrive at Venice Beach to the same scene, only this time it's inside the gym. With air pollution pouring in the open windows, folk gasp and puff, straining to drive the toxins to the furthest depths of their lungs. It's time to wake up. It's not roses you're smelling.

Monoxide Madness

Worst of it is, you can't smell the worst of it. Carbon monoxide for example, was a rare gas over the millions of years of human evolution. Consequently, the natural selection process which made us what we are today, had no way to select humans who were resistant to this poison. Our bodies can't even detect it. Carbon monoxide is odorless, tasteless, and invisible to all our body defenses.

When humans developed hemoglobin, in order to extract oxygen from the air, carbon monoxide wasn't around. The chemical make-up of the carbon monoxide we create today, by burning gas, oil and coal, just loves that hemoglobin mechanism. It combines with your hemoglobin 200 times more readily than oxygen. In preference to oxygen, your body sucks in every molecule of carbon monoxide in our urban air. It raises no protest, it can't even recognize carbon monoxide. The gas combines with your hemoglobin to form the deadly poison **carboxyhemoglobin**, and delivers it to every cell. That's why suicide by car exhaust is so popular. You die without even noticing.

Don't think you can dodge carbon monoxide, or any other toxic man-made gas. If you live in a major city in America, your blood levels of carboxyhemoglobin are likely to be **three times** that of folk in small mountain communities.[1,2] As an athlete you are in double jeopardy, because you use a lot more air than sedentary folk. And don't think it doesn't affect you. Vital capacity (VO_2 max) starts to decline at a blood level of carboxyhemoglobin of 2.6%, an average level found in non-smoking, sedentary, urban folk.[3]

The Central Park Lesson

But you're a lot tougher than couch potatoes - right? That's what I and a lot of athletes I worked with thought too. So you don't make the same mistake, here's our experience.

In the 1980s, I was doing research at Rockefeller University in New York. I trained with an enthusiastic group of runners in Central Park most evenings, and ran the New York Marathon three times and about 20 other marathons. As a good little scientist seeking to improve performance, I measured everything in our group, including lung function, heart function, lactic acidosis, anaerobic threshold, and VO₂ max. We improved regularly and ran marathons faster every year. We were typical examples of athletes slowly destroying their health and performance.

We failed to appreciate just how much your body becomes part of its usual environment. Finally I started to realize how the polluted air in Central Park was dosing us with lead, ozone, nitrogen disoxide, carbon monoxide, and a host of other poisons. My records show lung inflammation, bronchitis, and an incidence of upper respiratory tract infections much higher than the sedentary average.

Those of us who were determined to protect our health left New York. I went to San Diego permanently, and my health and running performance improved almost immediately. Those who went to the mountains to Boulder, Colorado, did best. They had the double advantage of cleaner air and training at the right altitude.

By running in the air pollution of New York, we had been violating a basic principle of sports nutrition. We were allowing, you might say encouraging, toxic chemicals to become part of our structure. If you train in an urban area now, think about it. For the best of health and strength it's time to leave.

I wrote up the New York data for **Runners World**, but they refused to publish it. After all, the New York Road Runners Club is one of the largest in the nation, and our findings might discourage city folk from running. It might also discourage them from buying all that running gear advertised in the magazine, but of course, that wasn't even a consideration.

Smart Olympic coaches know the score. They keep their athletes away from cities. Bob Sevene, coach of Joan Benoit Samuelson who won the women's marathon in Los Angeles in 1984 summed it up.

> "We'll arrive in Los Angeles on Friday, rest on Saturday, race on Sunday, and leave."[4]

If you want a long, healthy athletic career you'll do the same.

Getting Smoggier

The Environmental Protection Agency uses the Pollution Standard Index (PSI) to measure air pollution on a scale of 0 - 500. Zero to PSI 50 is near pure air. Above PSI 100 is, "unhealthy". Above PSI 200 is "hazardous to health." In defiance of America's shining Clean Air Act, New York now has more than 200 days per year above PSI 100. Los Angeles is even smoggier, with over 100 days above PSI 200, and growing worse by the year.

In February 1992, the US National Research Council reported, that the air quality in the Los Angeles Basin was the worst in the nation. Ten years later it is just as bad. It subjects the twelve million residents to lung disorders, damaged immunity, and a lifespan three years shorter than average. Indoors, even with windows closed, Los Angeles residents receive toxic doses of man-made pollutants while they sleep.[5]

Asthma Sounds The Warning

Dr Russell Sherwin and colleagues at the University of Southern California, recently examined the lungs of young Los Angeles residents aged 14-25, who had died in traffic accidents and homicides. They found severe damage, including chronic bronchitis, lung inflammation, and actual holes burned into the lung tissues by the air pollution.[6]

Burned lungs are bad news, but the strongest evidence of the health devastation caused by air pollution is the huge increase in asthma. Calling asthma "The epidemic in the absence of infection," a 1997 report in *Science*, the leading American science journal, documents that the incidence of asthma has **doubled** in the last 20 years.[7]

The implications of this man-made disease are devastating. Asthma is not only a severe illness itself, but, is even more important as a marker for systemic degeneration of the body. Asthma is an immune dysfunction, so any unnatural increase also signals a general decline in immunity **to all diseases**.

This immune decline is now so pervasive in America, that the US National Research Council instructed immunologists across the nation to redouble efforts to find a solution.[8] Ten years of effort so far, have produced nothing except a worsening of the problem. You cannot rely on government, nor on medicine. You have to learn to protect yourself.

Antioxidant Protection

Most air pollutants do their damage by oxidation. So, despite the lack of studies on athletes, it's a logical assumption that antioxidants should protect you some. It certainly works with animals. In one report, two groups of rats were exposed to 0.1 ppm of ozone in air, the level exceeded every day in New York and Los Angeles. One group was supplemented with high doses of vitamin E. The other was given vitamin E in the diet equivalent of the RDA for humans. Most of the RDA group developed lung lesions within two weeks. Over 80% of the high-dose vitamin E group remained healthy throughout the study.[9]

In another report, rats were given either 100 IU or 1,000 IU of vitamin E per kilogram of food, and exposed to 0.8 ppm of ozone (the high end of current levels in Los Angeles). The rats given the high-dose vitamin E were far better protected.[10]

For some unknown reason, athletes are reluctant to deliberately expose themselves to toxic gases to test antioxidant protection. Can't understand it myself, since they expose themselves every day on the freeway. Nevertheless scientists can't get subjects even for pay, and have to try and do it sideways. In one of the few human studies, Dr. E. Calabrese gave healthy volunteers 600 IU of vitamin E daily for four weeks. He then exposed their blood cells in vitro (in the test tube) to hydrogen peroxide, an oxidation product of air pollution. The pollutant crucified the cells. By the second week of supplementation however, the vitamin E afforded considerable protection.[11] If you have to be an urban dweller, don't leave home without it.

You will see ahead in the chapter on antioxidants, that vitamin E is only a small part of the air pollution answer. As an urban athlete seeking to excel, you need to don complete antioxidant armor every day to even partially save your breath. If you are really serious about your sport, plan your life to leave the cities permanently behind you.

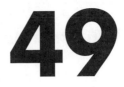

ANTIOXIDANT ARMOR

Every breath you take creates damaging residues of oxygen called **free radicals**.[1] In 1954 Denman Harmon at the University of Nebraska was the first to suggest that these microscopic nasties are *the* major cause of human aging.[2]

Since then many thousands of research papers have proven beyond doubt that free radical damage is a big part of the mechanism of more than 100 forms of degeneration of the flesh, including cardiovascular diseases, cancers, arthritis, diabetes, and many types of organ degeneration. From wrinkling of the skin and blindness to gastrointestinal, liver and kidney diseases, and destruction of the brain by Alzheimer's and Parkinson's, free radicals literally eat you alive. They are also a large component of the damage caused by exercise.[3-5]

Oxidation Is Essential

Sounds like an inescapable fate, and it is. We live by oxygen and we die by oxygen. In a miniscule nutshell here's how it happens. Energy from sunlight is stored in the food you eat. After digestion, the energy is transferred to your flesh by a complex process of electron transfer which creates your basic energy molecule, **adenosine triphosphate** (ATP).

This process bears little resemblance to the schoolboy story of the body burning calories to produce energy. Calories are a measure of the amount of heat produced when you burn food in a crude instrument called a bomb calorimeter. Your body is not a bomb calorimeter. It doesn't *burn* anything. It works by controlled nuclear power.

Unfortunately, the calorie fable, taught to children to keep things simple, has become a pervasive adult belief in Western Society. Even some dumbo health professionals still adhere to it. Causes endless problems for scientists trying to explain anything to the public about food, energy, or control of bodyfat.

Being highly profitable, the notion of calories also continues to bombard us from the media every day, cleverly touted by judas scientists in "official" white coats and faces, bolstered by EKGs and stethoscopes and other sacred symbols, selling everything from diet drugs, drinks and glop to equally useless cellulite creams, electrical zappers, and full rubber sweat suits in multiple designer colors. If you want to fully comprehend the perfidy of commerce, tap into the internet for pages of pharmaceutical advertising from only 40 - 50 years ago. The claims made then for useless glop and weird medical devices, (such as those shown above) seem laughable now. In a few years time so will those claims made by the same advertising today.

Transfer of the energy in carbohydrates, fats and proteins to ATP occurs by **controlled oxidation**. The metabolic residue of this process consists of pairs of hydrogen atoms which release from the food molecules (H_2) and combine with oxygen (O) delivered by the hemoglobin in your blood to make H_2O, pure water. For 95% of your oxygen consumption, energy production this process, called the **tetravalent reduction of oxygen with cytochrome C oxidase**, is clean as a fresh-washed baby's bum. Controlled oxidation is the basic process of human life.

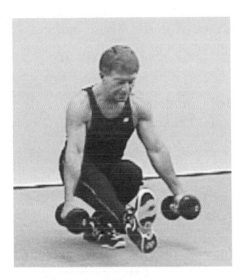

Michael Colgan demonstrating single leg squats from the Colgan Power Program.

Uncontrolled Oxidation

The remaining 5% of your oxygen is converted to energy by **univalent reduction**, which is dirtier than the bum before the bath. Many molecules of oxygen become unstable and leak out of the energy cycle. They become free radicals, damaging everything they touch. Left unattended they generate inflammation, pain, and all sorts of other mayhem.[4]

To get an idea how free radicals damage you, consider the well-tended babe. Each of the stable atoms that compose its bum, has electrons spinning around the nucleus in opposing pairs to balance their electromagnetic forces. Left undisturbed, neighboring atoms all spin along merrily, and the miraculous mosaic of flesh they compose remains healthy indefinitely.

But if the babe is neglected, atoms start to gain or lose single electrons. Their electromagnetic charges become unbalanced and they become free radicals. Seeking to restore that balance, which holds together not only the baby's bum but the whole fabric of the Universe, the free radicals either donate their extra electrons to, or steal electrons from, the nearest stable molecules of flesh. Those molecules then become free radicals, setting up a chain of free radical damage. The bum begins to develop a rash.

This process of **uncontrolled oxidation** is the largest single cause of degeneration known to science. The rusting of steel, the browning of a cut apple, the rotting of meat, and the decay of human flesh all occur primarily by uncontrolled oxidation. Even glass and granite rock eventually oxidize to dust.[5]

Exercise Multiplies Free Radicals

Exercise uses 12 – 20 times more oxygen than slumping in front of the tube,[6] which pushes uncontrolled oxidation into the stratosphere. Alexandre Quintanilha has demonstrated a three-fold increase in muscle free radicals with only moderate exercise.[7] And, in the early 1980s, he and Lester Packer at the University of California at Irvine were the first to show that free radicals generated by exercise cause extensive muscle damage.[8]

These free radicals come in numerous different types. Some last only fractions of a second, others continue creating damage long-term. The **semiquinone radical** from tobacco smoke for example, can remain active for days.[9] I'm betting that, as an athlete, you don't smoke or allow smokers around you, so you don't have to worry about that one. The main free radicals you should worry about are those increased by exercise. The worst of them are listed in the following table.

Table 8:
Major Free Radicals Increased By Exercise.

Radical	Chemical Symbol
Hydroxyl radical	$HO\bullet$
Alkoxyl radical	$RO\bullet$
Peroxyl radical	$ROO\bullet$
Hydrogen peroxide	H_2O_2
Superoxide anion radical	O_2-
Singlet oxygen	$^1O_2$
Nitric oxide radical	$NO\bullet$
Peroxynitrite	$ONOO-$

Sources: Colgan Institute, San Diego, 1998

Different Toxins: Different Antidotes

If you inject cobra anti-venom into someone bitten by a black mamba, it is powerless to prevent their death, because the poisons of the two snakes have different chemical structures. To defeat any strong toxin you have to use the anti-toxin specifically designed for the job.

The same applies to free radicals. The table shows that the major free radicals increased by exercise cover a wide range of chemical structures. Consequently, they need a wide range of specific antioxidants to defeat them. So whenever you see health media touting this or that flavor-of-the-month antioxidant as the only one you need, *don't believe them!*

Some antioxidants, such as grape seed extract are wide-spectrum and attack numerous free radicals, but with only moderate effect. Other antioxidants, such as Vitamin C, attack a few free radicals very strongly but don't even notice others.

The second big consideration in using antioxidants is the basic nutritional principle of synergy. We would all be dead of free radical damage tomorrow, were it not for the body's production of endogenous antioxidants, mainly superoxide dismutase, catalase, and glutathione. These antioxidants "quench" free radicals by receiving or donating an electron. Does this action not convert the antioxidant itself into a free radical? Yes it does, but thanks to the brilliant chemistry designed into the human body, other antioxidants immediately step in and quench it, and still others quench them. Eventually, this chemical chain ends up as harmless residues, mainly water and carbon dioxide, for use in other body chemistry or excretion via urine, sweat and breath.

With the intense training that is essential to excel in sport today, endogenous antioxidants alone cannot protect you. The sheer volume of oxygen used easily overwhelms your body's production of antioxidants. Worse, it also exhausts your store of cytochrome C, the vital chemical noted earlier that shunts oxygen through the clean tetravalent reduction pathway.[10] Consequently more of the oxygen gets shunted into the dirty univalent reduction pathway. So with any exercise beyond miniature golf, you get a double-whammy of free radicals.

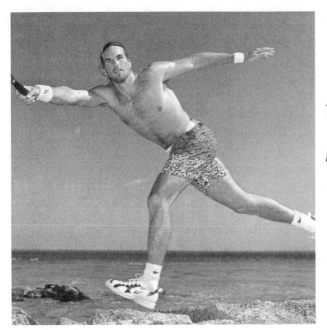

Tennis champion Australian Pat Rafter shows the grace of human form and movement that come with the right nutrition and training.

Supplementary Antioxidants To The Rescue

You can't just add cytochrome C to vitamin supplements as some manufacturers have done. There's not a shred of evidence that oral supplements can increase muscle cell cytochrome C by a molecule. The same goes for all those bogus supplements of superoxide dismutase and catalase. Only glutathione works by mouth and not very well at that.[11] Taking precursors of glutathione, such as n-acetyl cysteine is a better bet.

In the event of cytochrome C depletion, which occurs in all strenuous activity beyond a few minutes duration, the only nutrient we know that can pinch-hit for it is **coenzyme Q10 (CoQ10)**. To assist in use of oxygen, the muscles of highly trained athletes learn to produce much higher levels of CoQ10 than muscles of sedentary folk.[12,13] You can achieve similar high levels by taking CoQ10 supplements.[14]

One caution. In doubling for cytochrome C, CoQ10 itself produces the particularly nasty type of free radical called **superoxide anion radicals**. Unless quenched, these bad boys quickly create their own chain of damage.[15]

During the long training necessary to increase muscle CoQ10 naturally, it's likely that the muscles of athletes also put in place all the other antioxidants necessary to neutralize the superoxide radicals created by CoQ10. Taking CoQ10 by mouth, however, puts nothing else in place to deal with its superoxide radicals and, by itself, may *increase* free radical damage. Yes, taking a single antioxidant such as CoQ10 may *increase* free radical damage.

Vitamin E Whacks Superoxide But . . .

Vitamin E can come to the rescue. Inside the protective fatty membrane that surrounds each muscle cell, just climbing a flight of stairs looses a flood of free radicals, including singlet oxygen, hydrogen peroxide, and superoxide radicals like those produced by CoQ10. These oxidize the living fat of the membrane, that is, destroy the fat by turning it rancid, a form of damage called **lipid peroxidation**. The rancid fat then continues the chain of damage as **peroxyl radicals**. Over a period of days they inflame and often kill affected cells.[16] Peroxyl radicals are one reason that the muscles of athletes are often more painful the second day, rather than the first day, after an intense workout.

Fat-soluble antioxidant vitamin E, quenches a lot of the lipid peroxidation that starts this chain of damage. But in doing so, it becomes a pro-oxidant, producing damaging **tocopherol radicals** and **tocopheroxyl radicals**. Al Tappel of the University of California, Davis, was the first to show that **vitamin C** has to step in to quench these nasties, and regenerate the vitamin E.[17] This action requires a lot of supplementary vitamin C, without which vitamin E supplements may cause more harm than good.

Selenium Too

Of course, your body doesn't rely on vitamin E alone. Vitamin E works in synergy with the endogenous antioxidant glutathione to quench lipid peroxidation. But to do so, glutathione needs the mineral **selenium**, which "holds" the lipid radicals so that glutathione can get a crack at them.[18] Selenium is also required for vitamin E to function properly.[18]

It's not much use, however, taking selenium, if you don't have enough glutathione in the first place. Intense exercise can deplete muscle glutathione by 40%, and liver glutathione (from which the muscles get their refills) by 80%.[19] So you better be taking preformed glutathione too, or its precursor **n-acetyl cysteine**, both of which work in different ways to increase body glutathione levels.[20,21]

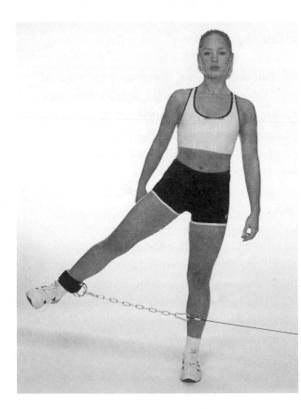

Melissa Canales demonstrates a cable abduction exercise from the Colgan Power Program.

So Far You Need . . .

Let's take stock. Already we need supplementary CoQ10, vitamin E, vitamin C, selenium, glutathione, and n-acetyl cysteine to combat the free radical damage caused by exercise. And the list has hardly begun.

I've deliberately sketched these few examples of a tiny corner of the free radical circus, to demonstrate four principles of antioxidant use.

1. There are numerous different types of free radicals. Some are quenched by one antioxidant, some by another.

2. Antioxidants work in synergy with each other. Dumping arbitrary amounts of one or other antioxidant into your body may disrupt that synergy to create a pro-oxidant situation, that is, may *increase* your free radical burden, not reduce it.

3. Before you take any antioxidant to combat free radical damage, you better know the main complementary antioxidants necessary to support its use, and take them also.

4. You better know how much of each antioxidant to take to maintain the synergistic balance between them.

More Antioxidants

Vitamin A is an essential nutrient which should form part of your basic daily vitamin/mineral supplement. But doses of vitamin A above 10,000 IU, can accumulate over time to toxic levels. Your body can make *some* vitamin A from **beta-carotene**, which, because it is virtually non-toxic, has become a popular supplement source for vitamin A.

The antioxidant function of beta-carotene, however, is independent of its role as a precursor of vitamin A.[22] Beta-carotene neutralizes singlet oxygen radicals very nicely,[23] and does so better than vitamin C or vitamin E.[24] This action alone warrants its inclusion in a sports antioxidant supplement. **Lycopene**, the analogue of beta-carotene, found plentifully in tomatoes, is even better. It is best known as a major protector of the human eye from oxidation by ultra-violet light. But it also has greater capacity than other carotenoids to quench singlet oxygen radicals.[25]

The oxy-carotenoids, notably **lutein** and **zeaxanthin** also protect the eyes, and other tissues from oxidation by a variety of mechanisms. They are especially important for athletes who train outdoors and are subject to large amounts of ultra-violet. In Australia and northern New Zealand where holes in the ozone layer have increased ultra-violet exposure, lutein and zeaxanthin are essential to protect the eyes.

Carotenoids also work with vitamin E, selenium, and glutathione to inhibit peroxyl radicals, thus helping to prevent lipid peroxidation of cell membranes.[26] So to gain the best antioxidant protection for athletes, we have to add beta-carotene and lycopene to the mix, and probably lutein and zeaxanthin also.

Mineral Antioxidants

We've looked at the cell membrane, where the antioxidant mineral selenium works. Now we'll take a peek inside the cell at more antioxidant minerals. In this short account I have room to discuss only one villain of the free radical circus, so I'll focus on superoxide radicals.

In the body of the cell, the endogenous antioxidant, superoxide dismutase (SOD), is king. SOD "sucks" the extra electron from superoxide radicals, thereby producing hydrogen peroxide radicals. Glutathione, or the other main endogenous antioxidant, catalase, then converts the hydrogen peroxide into harmless oxygen and water.

To do this trick they need essential minerals. The sucker on SOD is made of **copper**, and SOD also requires the mineral **zinc** to keep it stable. As we saw above, glutathione requires both **selenium** and the amino acid cysteine. Catalase requires both **iron** and **copper** in order to do its work. So now we have to add the minerals iron, copper, and zinc to the selenium already included in the antioxidant mix.

Manganese Too

The mitochondria of your cells are mechanisms that evolved from symbiotic bacteria millions of years ago. They convert all fuel to energy in the body. This frantic activity also produces the bulk of your free radicals, especially those caused by exercise.[27] Nearly 50 years ago Denman Harman at the University of Nebraska proposed the oxidation theory of cell damage. He was dead right.[5] Since then we have learned that free radical damage to the mitochondria, especially by superoxide radicals, causes most of the decline in human performance that occurs with age, and, likely, also determines human lifespan.[28,29]

Thus, your mitochondria need potent antioxidant protection. The clean-up squad of glutathione and catalase remain unchanged, but

SOD takes a stronger form. Mitochondrial SOD uses the essential mineral **manganese** to suck the unstable electron from superoxide radicals. So manganese is another important mineral addition to sports antioxidants.

Alpha-Lipoic Acid

A bunch of popular articles are calling **alpha-lipoic acid** the "newest", the "best", the "master," the "universal" antioxidant, as if it is more important than all the rest.[30,31] Don't be fooled. It's neither new nor universal, just another cog in the wheel.

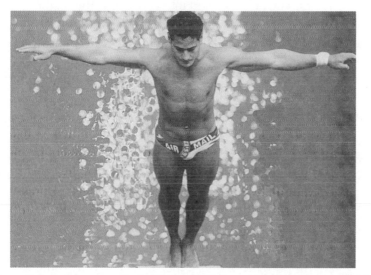

Greg Louganis, greatest diver of all time, about to take flight.

Discovered in the human body in 1951, for 30 years alpha-lipoic acid was thought to be a simple co-enzyme in the energy cycle. Meanwhile, some researchers found it could prevent scurvy in guinea pigs deliberately made deficient in vitamin C. (Like humans, guinea pigs are one of the few mammals that lack the liver enzyme necessary for their bodies to make vitamin C.) Alpha-lipoic acid also corrected vitamin E deficiency in rats. These findings suggested that it might have widespread antioxidant activity in both water (vitamin C) and lipid (vitamin E) environments.[32]

Starting in the mid-'80s, a rapid and ongoing series of studies spearheaded by Lester Packer, one of the world's top experts in antioxidants, showed that alpha-lipoic acid can directly neutralize singlet oxygen radicals, hydroxyl radicals, and some peroxyl radicals. Its metabolite, **dihydrolipoic acid**, also neutralizes peroxynitrite radicals, particularly nasty gremlins that contain both oxygen and nitrogen radicals.[33-36]

In addition, alpha-lipoic acid helps to regenerate vitamin C, vitamin E, glutathione and probably CoQ10.[33-36] It's a very busy molecule in the human body. Exposing the fallacy that it is the "master" or "universal" antioxidant, however, the same research shows that alpha-lipoic acid cannot neutralize hydrogen peroxide or most superoxide radicals.[32-36] Athletes taking alpha-lipoic acid as their sole source of nutrient antioxidants, would quickly put their bodies into a sorry state of free radical damage.

Alpha-Lipoic Acid For Athletes

Dr. Lester Packer's research[33] indicates that your body does not make enough of alpha-lipoic acid for stressful situations such as exercise. And the body's ability to make it declines rapidly with usual aging. So athletes can benefit from a higher intake than couch potatoes.

These are important findings, because the only potent dietary source is red meats. In previous books and articles, I have documented how even drug-free red meats are not good food, both because of their high saturated fat content, and their high content of pro-inflammatory **arachidonic acid**.[37]

In order to take advantage of alpha-lipoic acid, the sensible strategy is to take it as a supplement. To do so safely, you should know that recent studies have revealed numerous other functions of this versatile nutrient, independent of its antioxidant action. It helps prevent protein degradation, chelates the toxic metals mercury and cadmium, improves learning and memory, and enhances insulin metabolism.[33,38-41]

All these functions have relevance for health, but that's a whole other story. I mention them only because the last item, insulin metabolism, bears directly on safety and dosage. You can easily take too much alpha-lipoic acid and become hypoglycemic.[33] Don't use this supplement at all if you have hypoglycemic tendencies. With athletes whose insulin is stable, at the Colgan Institute we use 100-400 mg of alpha-lipoic acid per day. That's about half the dose range used in successful studies of diabetic neuropathy, the approved use in Europe for this versatile nutrient.[33]

All the antioxidants covered in this chapter are included as part of the nutrient list in Chapter 1. To help athletes decide where their personal requirements might fit in the ranges of nutrients we use six criteria:

1. Exercise amount per week
2. Exercise Intensity
3. Bodyweight
4. Bodyfat
5. Age
6. Level of pollution in the living environment

From the table ahead score one point for each **low** category, two points for each **medium** category, three points for each **high** category. Add the scores to get your Daily Antioxidant Score, then apply it to the list of antioxidants given ahead.

Table 9:
Criteria to Obtain Daily Antioxidant Score

Criterion	Low (Score 1)	Medium (Score 2)	High (Score 3)
Training Duration (hours per week)	1-6	7-14	15-30
Training Intensity (dominant level VO₂ max)	40-50	60-70	70+
Bodyweight	80-150 lbs 36-68 kgs	151-220 lbs 68.5-100 kgs	220+ lbs 100+ kgs
Bodyfat (%) Male Female	Below 10% Below 15%	11-16% 16-20%	17%+ 22%+
Age	Below 30	31-45	45+
Pollution Levels (where you live & train)	Mountains, rural clean	Suburban	Urban

Source: ©Colgan Institute, 1997

For example, take a male who trains 10 hours a week (score 2), at 70% + of VO₂ max (score 3), who weighs 200 lbs (score 2), and is below 10 % bodyfat (score 1), is below 30 years of age (score 1), and lives in a clean mountain environment (score 1). His total Daily Antioxidant Score is 10, so his antioxidant supplement is listed in the 10-12 column of Table 10.

Some important rules. Always begin an antioxidant program at the lowest end of the scale shown, that is, the first column (6-9) of Table 10. Then gradually work up to your ideal daily mix over a period of six months. This working time is essential for your body to grow the necessary enzymes and other chemicals to deal with all these concentrated nutrients. Otherwise you are asking for unpleasant reactions that can ***prevent*** your body from using the nutrients. Also, most of them will end up as expensive urine.

Even after your body has adapted to the enriched nutrient environment, do not exceed the amounts given by your Daily Antioxidant Score. And if your score declines, say because you cut your exercise volume, then reduce your antioxidant intake accordingly. Divide your antioxidant mix into three, and take it always with food, preferably breakfast, lunch, and dinner. Do not take antioxidants without food.

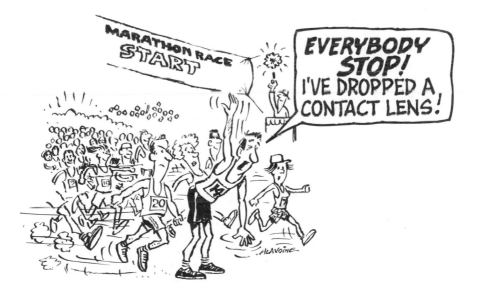

Table 10:
Daily Antioxidant Mix used with Athletes*

Antioxidant Nutrient	Daily Score			
	6-9	10-12	13-15	16-18
Vitamin E (IU)** (D-alpha-tocopherol succinate)+	400	800	1200	1600
Vitamin C (gm) (Ascorbic acid, mixed mineral ascorbates, ascorbyl palmitate)	1.0	2.0	3.0	4.0
Beta-carotene (IU)**	10,000	20,000	35,000	50,000
Coenzyme Q10 (mg)	30	50	75	1000
L-glutathione (mg)	50	100	150	200
N-acetyl cysteine (gm)++	100	200	300	400
Selenium (mcg) (L-selenomethionne),	200	300	450	600
Iron (mg) (Iron picolinate)	10	16	25	30
Zinc (mg) (Zinc picolinate)	15	25	35	50
Copper (mg) (Copper gluconate)	0.5	1.25	2.0	3.0
Manganese (mg) (Manganese gluconate)	5	10	20	30
Alpha-lipoic acid (mg)	100	200	300	400
Lycopene (mg)	20	40	70	100
Lutein (mg)	10	20	35	50
Rutin, hesperidin, naringin (mg) (mixed citrus flavonoids)	200	300	400	500
Procyanidins (mg) (grape seed extract, standardized to 95%)	100	125	160	200
Catechins (mg) (green tea extracts, standardized to 20%)	10	20	30	40
Bilobetin, amentoflavones (mg) (ginkgo biloba extract, standardized to 24%)	8	12	16	20
Silymarin, taxifolin (mg) (milk thistle extract, standardized to 80%)	50	100	150	200
Genestein, diadzein (mg) (soybean isoflavone extract, standardized to 10%)	10	20	60	100
Anthocyanins (mg) (bilberry extract, standardized to 25%)	10	15	20	25
Melatonin (mg)	1.0	2.0	3.0	4.0

** *I,U, International Units are obsolete measures no longer used in nutrition science. But, because they continue to appear on most supplement labels, they are used here for your convenience.*

+*Preferred forms of nutrients used by the Colgan Institute are given, because different forms of the same nutrient have widely different absorption rates and degrees of efficacy. The figures cannot be applied to other forms.*

++*N-acetyl cysteine should be used only in conjunction with at least three times the amount of vitamin C. Otherwise n-acetyl cysteine can precipitate as cysteine in the kidneys and possibly cause kidney stones in sensitive individuals.*

*Source: ©Colgan Institute, 1998

50

GOING FOR THE GUSTO!

As noted earlier 99.9% of your body is made of gaseous liquid, and solid mineral elements. If you want to function optimally you have to get your mineral nutrition right first before you consider anything else. Then you have to get all the vitamins right and the appropriate adjunctive nutrients. I have tried to give you the latest science to enable you to accomplish this task.

You can see, however, that research on optimal intakes of minerals, vitamins and other nutrients and on nutrient status of humans still has a long way to go. The Colgan Institute has spent the last 27 years doing nutritional research and analyses, and nutrition programs for more than 36,000 people. The levels of supplementation we use and the forms of nutrients we use today are the best effort result of that work.

As with all science, I urge you to examine the research references yourself before deciding to adopt anything from our program. And if you do adopt anything, it is done without our supervision, and therefore entirely at your own choice and risk. You can and should consult the medical references given for each chapter on the Internet, in the US National Medical Library at http//igm.nlm.nih.gov/.

Optimal nutrition is a neverending story. We will continue to progress and to inform you of our discoveries. You can e-mail us anytime at **team@colganinstitute.com.**

And you can also attend our four-day Sports Nutrition Intensives given periodically in various beautiful places all over the Earth, and listed on our websites: www.colganinstitute.com, www.colgansemi-nars.com, and www.colganpowerprogram.com.

Go for all the gusto of life, and may the twin contemporary gods of Science and Nature bless your efforts to perform *celtius, altius, fortius.*

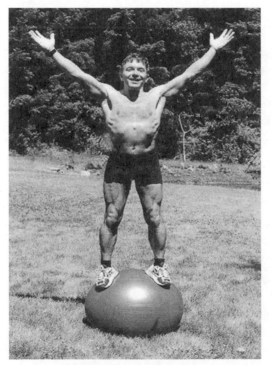

Going for the gusto!

REFERENCES

Introduction

1. Colgan M. **Optimum Sports Nutrition**. New York, Advanced Research Press, 1993.
2. **Recommended Dietary Allowances, Tenth Edition**. Washington DC: National Academy Press, 1989.
3. Harper AE. Official dietary allowances: those pesky RDAs. **Nutrition Today**, 1974;9:15-25.
4. Manore MM. Effects of physical activity on thiamine, riboflavin, and vitamin B-6 requirements. **Am J Clin Nutr**, 2000;72:598S-606S.
5. Weaver CM. Calcium requirements of physically active people. **Am J Clin Nutr**, 2000;72.579S-584S.
6. Maughan RJ. Role of micronutrients in sport and physical activity. **Br Med Bull**, 1999;55:683-690.
7. Dwyer J. Old wine in new bottles? The RDA and the DRI. **Nutrition**, 2000;16:488-492.
8. Johnson RK, Kennedy E. The 2000 Dietary Guidelines for Americans: what are the changes and why were they made? The Dietary Guidelines Advisory Committee. **J Am Diet Assoc**, 2000;100:769-774.
9. Kant AK. Consumption of energy-dense, nutrient-poor foods by adult Americans: nutritional and health implications. The third national health and nutrition examination survey, 1988-1994[In Process Citation]. **Am J Clin Nutr**, 2000;72:929-936.
10. Seidell JC. Obesity, insulin resistance and diabetes – a worldwide epidemic. **Br J Nutr**, 2000;83:S5-S8.
11. Stang J, et al. Relationships between vitamin and mineral supplement use, dietary intake, and dietary adequacy among adolescents. **J Am Diet Assoc**, 2000;100:905-910.

Chapter 1

1. Lovelock J. **The Ages of Gaia: A Biography of the Living Earth**. New York NY: WW Norton, 1988.

Chapter 2

1. Johnson RK, Kennedy E. The 2000 Dietary Guidelines for Americans: what are the changes and why were they made? The Dietary Guidelines Advisory Committee. **J Am Diet Assoc**, 2000;100:769-774.

2.   Colgan M. **Optimum Sports Nutrition**. New York, Advanced Research Press, 1993.
3.   **Recommended Dietary Allowances, Tenth Edition**. Washington DC: National Academy Press, 1989.
4.   Dwyer J. Old wine in new bottles? The RDA and the RDI. **Nutrition**, 2000;16:488-492.
5.   Harper AE. Official dietary allowances: those pesky RDAs. **Nutrition Today**, 1974;9:15-25.
6.   Colgan M. **The New Nutrition**. Vancouver, Apple Publishing, 1995.
7.   Oakley GP. Eat right and take a multivitamin. **New Engl J Med**, 1998;338:1060-1061.
8.   Krumbach CJ, et al. A report of vitamin and mineral supplement use among university athletes in a division I institution. **Int J Sport Nutr**, 1999;9:416-425.
9.   Arsenault J, Kennedy J. Dietary supplement use in US Army Special Operations candidates. **Mil Med**, 1999;164:495-501.
10.   Lyle BJ, et al. Supplement users differ from nonusers in demographic, lifestyle, dietary and health characteristics. **J Nutr**, 1998;128:2355-2362.
11.   Constantini NW, et al. Iron status of highly active adolescents: evidence of depleted iron stores in gymnasts. **Int J Sport Nutr Exerc Metab**, 2000;10:62-70.
12.   Ziegler PJ, et al. Nutritional and physiological status of US national figure skaters. **Int J Sport Nutr**, 1999;9:345-360.
13.   Ronsen O, et al. Supplement use and nutritional habits in Norwegian elite athletes. **Scand J Med Sci Sports**, 1999;9:28-35.
14.   Nuviala RJ. Magnesium, zinc, and copper status in women involved in different sports. **Int J Sport Nutr**, 1999;9:295-309.
15.   **Recommended Dietary Allowances, Seventh Edition**. Washington, DC: National Academy of Sciences, 1968.
16.   **Recommended Dietary Allowances, Ninth Edition**. Washington, DC: National Academy of Sciences, 1980.
17.   Duffield AJ, Thomson CD. A comparison of methods of assessment of dietary selenium intakes in Otago, New Zealand. **Br J Nutr**, 1999;82:131-138.
18.   Williams RJ. Pantothenic acid – a vitamin. **Science**, 1939;89:486.
19.   Wolinsky I, Driscoll JA, (Eds). **Sports Nutrition**. London: CRC Press, 1997.
20.   Colgan M. Reported in: Wolinsky I, Driscoll JA, (Eds). **Sports Nutrition**. London: CRC Press, 1997.
21.   Walsh NP, et al. Glutamine, exercise and immune function. Links and possible mechanisms. **Sports Med**, 1998;26:177-191.
22.   Schroder H, et al. Nutrition antioxidant status and oxidative stress in professional basketball players: effects of a three compound antioxidative supplement. **Int J Sports Med**, 2000;21:146-150.
23.   Shephard RJ, Shek PN. Immunological hazards from nutritional imbalance in athletes. **Exerc Immunol Rev**, 1998;4:22-48
24.   Jonnalagadda SS, et al. Energy and nutrient intakes of the United States

National Women's Artistic Gymnastics Team. **Int J Sport Nutr**, 1998;8:331-344.

25. Ziegler PJ, et al. Nutritional and physiological status of US national figure skaters. **Int J Sport Nutr**, 1999;9:345-360.

26. Ronsen O, et al. Supplement use and nutritional habits in Norwegian elite athletes. **Scand J Med Sci Sports**, 1999;9:28-35.

27. Sugiura K, et al. Nutritional intake of elite Japanese track-and-field athletes. **Int J Sports Nutr**, 1999;9:202-212.

28. Ames BN. Micronutrient deficiencies. A major cause of DNA damage. **Ann N Y Acad Sci**, 1999;889:87-106.

29. Gross P, Marti B. Risk of degenerative ankle joint disease in volleyball players: study of former elite athletes. **Int J Sports Med**, 1999;20:58-63.

30. Marti B, Knobloch M. Subjective health and career status of former top athletes. A controlled 15-year follow-up study. **Schweiz Z Sportmed**, 1991;39:125-131.

31. Tucker A. Delayed damage to the hip joint in competitive sports. **Radiologe**, 1990;30:497-500.

32. Marti B, et al. Is excessive running predictive of degenerative hip disease? Controlled study of former elite athletes. **BMJ**, 1989;299:91-93.

33. Tysvaer AT, et al. Head and neck injuries among Norwegian soccer players. A neurological, electroencephalographic, radiologic and neuropsychological evaluation. **Tidsskr Nor Laegeforen**, 1992;112:1268-1271.

34. McKenzie JE, et al. Comparative investigation of neurofibrillary damage in the temporal lobe in Alzheimer's disease, Down's syndrome and dementia pugilistica. **Neurodegeneration**, 1996;5:259-264.

Chapter 3

1. Carson, R. **Silent Spring**. New York, NY: Houghton, Mifflin Co, 1962.

2. Jenson AA. Polychlorinated bipheryls (PCBs) and polychlorodibenso-p-dioxins in human milk, blood and adipose tissue. **Sci Total Environ**, 1987, 64:259-293.

3. Noren K, Meironyte D. Certain organochlorine contaminants in Swedish human milk in perspective of the past 20-30 years. **Chemosphere**, 2000;40:111-1123.

4. Kitabchi AE, et al. Specific receptor sites for alpha-tcocpherol in purified isolated adrenocortical cell membrane. **Biochem Biophys Res Comm**, 1980;96:1739-46.

5. Lazarou J. et al. Incidence of adverse drug reactions in hospitalized patents: A meta analysis, **J Amer Assoc,** 1998;279:1200-1205.

Chapter 6

1. Colgan M. **The New Nutrition: Medicine for the Millennium.** Vancouver: Apple Publishing, 1994.
2. Trowell HC, Burkitt DP. **Western Disease.** New York, NY: Harvard University Press, 1981.
3. **USDA Publication No. 252.** Hyattsville MD: USDA, 1992.
4. Graci S. **The Power of Superfoods.** Scarborough, Canada: Prentice Hall, 1997.
5. Colgan M. **Optimum Sports Nutrition.** New York, NY: Advanced Research Press, 1993.
6. Colgan M. **Hormonal Health.** Vancouver: Apple Publishing, 1996.
7. Brand-Miller JC. Importance of glycemic index in diabetes. **Amer J Clin Nutr,** 1994;59:747S-752S.
8. Walberg Rankin J. Glycemic index and exercise metabolism. **Sports Science Exchange,** 1997;64:1-14: fred.net/ultrunr/glycemic.html.
9. Foster-Powerll K, Brand-Miller JC. International tables of glycemic index. **Amer J Clin Nutr,** 1995;62:871S-893S.
10. Jenkins DJ, et al. Metabolic effects of a low glycemic index diet. **Amer J Clin Nutr,** 1987;46:968-975.

Chapter 8

1. **National Research Council Recommended Dietary Allowances, Tenth Edition.** Washington, DC: National Academy Press, 1989.
2. Avioli LV. Calcium and osteoporosis. **Ann Rev Nutr,** 1984;4:471.
3. Stang J, et al. Relationship between vitamin and mineral supplement use, dietary intake and dietary adequacy among adolescents. J Am Dietet Assoc, 2000;100:905-910.
4. Rucinski A. Relationship of body image and dietary intake of competitive ice skaters. **J Am Dietet Assoc,** 1989;89:58-63.
5. Jonalagadda SS, et al. Energy and nutrient intakes of the United States Women's Artistic Gymnastics Team. **Int J Sports Med,** 1998;8:331-344.
6. Ziegler PJ, et al. Nutritional and physiological status of US national figure skaters. **Int J Sports Med**, 1999;9:345-360.
7. Sibtain M. Gastrointestinal absorption of calcium from milk and calcium salts. **New Engl J Med**, 1987;317:532.
8. Weaver CM. Calcium requirements of physically active people. **Am J Clin Nutr**, 2000;72(Suppl):579S-584S.
9. Lane NE, et al. Long-distance running bone density and osteoporosis. **J Am Med Assoc**, 1986;255:1147.
10. Hegsted M, et al. Urinary calcium and calcium balance in young men as affected by level of protein and phosphorus intake. **J Nutr,** 1981;111:553.
11. Petterson L, et al. Low bone mass density at multiple skeletal sites, including the appendicular skeleton in amenorrhic runners. **Calcif Tissue Int,**

1999;64:117-125.

12. Suominen H. Bone mineral density and long-term exercise: an average of cross-sectional athlete studies. **Sports Med**, 1993;16:316-330.

13. Hetland ML, et al. Low bone mass and high bone turnover in male long-distance runners. **J Clin Endocrin Metab**, 1993;77:770-773.

14. Warren MP, Stichl AL. Exercise and female adolescents effects on the reproductive and skeletal systems. **J Am Med Womans Assoc**, 1999;54:115-120.

15. Loucks AB, et al. Alterations in the hypothalamic-pituitary-ovarian axes in athletic women. **J Clin Endocrin Metab**, 1989;68:402-411.

16. De Souza MJ, et al. Effects of exercise training on sex steroids: endocrine profiles and clinical implications. **Infert Repr Med Clin North Amer**, 1992;3:129-148.

17. Brown M, et al. Hormone replacement therapy does not augment gain in muscle strength or fat-free mass in response to weight bearing exercise. **J Gerontol**, 1997;32:B168-B170.

18. Hackney AC, et al. Hypothalamic-pituitary-testicular function in endurance trained males. **Int J Sports Med**, 1990;34:949-954.

19. Arce JC, et al. Exercise and male factor infertility. **Sports Med**, 1992;15:146-149.

20. Rico H, et al. Body composition in post pubertal boy cyclists. **J Sports Med Phys Fitness**, 1993;33:278-281.

21. Colgan M. **The New Nutrition: Medicine For The Millennium.** Vancouver: Apple Publishing, 1995

22. Chu JY, et al. Integumentary loss of calcium. **Am J Clin Nutr**, 1979;32:1699-1702.

23. Charles P, et al. Dermal, intestinal and renal obligatory loss of calcium: relation to skeletal calcium loss. **Am J Clin Nutr**, 1991;54(Suppl):266S-272S.

24. Kiesges RC, et al. Changes in bone mineral content in male athletes. **J Amer Med Assoc**, 1996;276:226-230.

25. Bodwell CE, Erdman JW, (eds). **Nutrient Interactions**. New York: Marcel Dekker, 1988.

Chapter 9

1. **National Research Council Recommended Dietary Allowances, Tenth Edition.** Washington, DC: National Academy Press, 1989.

2. Chasiotis D. Role of cyclic AMP and inorganic phosphate in the regulation of glycogenolysis during exercise. **Med Sci Sports Exerc**, 1988;20:545-550.

3. Ljinghall S, et al. Plasma potassium and phosphate concentration: influence by adrenalin infusion beta blockade and physical exercise. **Acta Medica Scand**, 1987;221:83-93.

4. Dale G, et al. Fitness, unfitness and phosphate. **Brit Med J**, 1987;294:939.

5. Clarkson PM, Haymes EM. Exercise and mineral status of athletes: calcium, magnesium, phosphorus and iron. **Med Sci Sports Exerc**, 1995;27:831-843.

6. Kreider RB, et al. Effects of phosphate loading on oxygen uptake, ventilato-

ry threshold and in performance. **Med Sci Sports Exerc,** 1990;22:250-255.

7.   Miller GW, et al. Effects of phosphate loading on anaerobic threshold. **Med Sci Sports Exerc**, 1991;23:S35.

8.   Stewart I, McNaughton L. Phosphate loading and effects on V02 max in trained cyclists. **Res Quart,** 1990;61:80-84.

9.   Cade R, et al. Effects of phosphate loading on 2-3-diphosphoglycerate and maximal oxygen uptake. **Med Sci Sports Exerc**, 1984;16:263-268.

10. Krieder RB, et al Effect of phosphate loading on metabolic and myocardial responses to maximal and endurance exercise. **Int J Sports Nutr,** 1992;2:20-47.

Chapter 10

1.   **Sodium: Potassium Ratios In Common Foods, Second Edition.** San Diego: The Colgan Institute, 1995.

2.   **National Research Council Recommended Dietary Allowances, Tenth Edition.** Washington, DC: National Academy Press, 1989.

3.   US National Research Council. Report of the Committee on Diet and Health. Washington DC: National Academy Press, 1989.

4.   Zorbas VG, et al. Potassium loading effect on potassium balance in athletes during prolonged restriction of muscular activity. **Biol Trace Elem Res,** 1999;70:1-19.

5.   McKenna MJ, et al. Effects of training on potassium, calcium, and hydrogen ion regulation in skeletal muscle and blood during exercise. **Acta Physiol Scand**, 1996;156:335-346.

6.   Knochel JP. Potassium deficiency during training in the heat. In Milvery P, (ed). **The Marathon.** New York: New York Academy of Sciences; 1977:175

7.   Short SH, Short WR. Four year study of university athletes' dietary intake. **J Amer Dietet Assoc,** 1983;82:632.

8.   Tarnopolsky MA, et al. Mixed carbohydrate supplementation increases carbohydrate oxidation and endurance exercise performance and alleviates potassium accumulation. **Int J Sport Nutr,** 1996;6:323-336.

Chapter 11

1.   **National Research Council Recommended Dietary Allowances, Tenth Edition.** Washington, DC: National Academy Press, 1989.

2.   Grimble RF, Grimble GK. Immunonutrition: role of sulfur amino acids, related amino acids and polyamines. **Nutrition,** 1998;4:605-610.

3.   Lyons J, et al. Blood glutathione synthesis rates in healthy adults receiving a sulfur amino acid-free diet. **Prac Natl Acad Sci, USA**, 200;97:5071-5076.

4.   Selhut J. Homocysteine metabolism. **Ann Rev Nutr,** 1999;19:217-246.

5.   Colgan M. **Beat Arthritis.** Vancouver: Apple Publishing, 2000.

6.   Raguso CA, et al. Cysteine kinetics and oxidation at different intakes of methionine and cysteine in young adults. **Am J Clin Nutr**, 2000;71:491-499.

Chapter 12

1.   DeSanto NG, et al. A contribution to the history of common salt. **Kidney Int Suppl,** 1997;59:S127-S134.
2.   DeSanto NG, et al.   Salt: a sacred substance.   **Kidney Int Suppl,** 1997;62:S111-S120.
3.   Arguelles J, et al. Adult offspring long-term effects of high salt and water intake during pregnancy. **Horm Behav,** 2000;37:156-162.
4.   Wilson DK, et al. The prevalence of salt sensitivity in an African-American adolescent population. **Ethn Dis,** 1999;9:350-358.
5.   Kulkarni S, et al. Stress and hypertension. WMJ, 1998;97:34-38.
6.   de Wardener HE. Sodium and hypertension. **Arch Mal Cocur Vaiss,** 1996;89 Spec No 4:9-15
7.   Sica DA. What are the influences of salt, potassium, the sympathetic nervous system, and the renin-angiotensin system on the circadian variation in blood pressure? **Blood Press Monit,** 1999;4 Suppl 2:S9-S16.
8.   Ljungman S. The Kidney as a Target of Hypertension. **Curr Hypertens Rep,** 1999;1:164-169.
9.   MacGregor GA. Nutrition and blood pressure. **Nutr Metab Cardiovasc Dis,** 1999;9(4 Suppl):6-15
10.   Fodor JG, et al. Lifestyle modification to prevent and control hypertension. 5. Recommendations on dietary salt. Canadian Hypertension Society, Canadian Coalition for High Blood Pressure Prevention and Control, Laboratory Centre for Disease Control at Health Canada, Heart and Stroke Foundation of Canada. **CMAJ,** 1999;160(9 Suppl):S29-S34.
11.   Kokkinos PF, Papademetriou V. Exercise and hypertension. **Coron Artery Dis,** 2000;11:99-102.

Chapter 13

1.   Wester PO. Magnesium. **Am J Clin Nutr,** 1987;45:1305-1312.
2.   Altura J, et al. (eds). Magnesium in **Cellular Processes and Medicine,** Basel: Karger, 1987.
3.   **National Research Council Recommended Dietary Allowances, Tenth Edition.** Washington, DC: National Academy Press, 1989.
4.   Dietary Reference Intakes. **Nutr Rev,** 1997;55:319-326.
5.   Yates AA, et al. Dietary Reference Intakes: the new basis for recommendations for calcium and related nutrients, B vitamins and choline. **J Am Diet Assoc,** 1998;98:699-706.
6.   Ford ES. Serum magnesium and ischaemic heart disease: findings from a

national sample of US adults. **Int J Epidemiol,** 1999;28:645-651.

7.   Steen SN, McKinney S. Nutrition assessment of college wrestlers. **Physician and Sports Med,** 1986;14:100.

8.   Bazarre TL, et al. Incidence of poor nutritional status among triathletes, endurance athletes and controls. **Med Sci Sports Exerc,** 1986;18(Suppl):S90.

9.   Jonalagadda SS, et al. Energy and nutrient intakes of the United States National Women's Gymnastics Team. **Int J Sports Nutr,** 1998;8:331-344.

10. Ziegler PJ, et al. Nutritional and physiological status of US National figure skaters. **Int J Sports Nutr,** 1999;9:345-360.

11. Buchman AL, et al. The effect of a marathon run on plasma and urine mineral and metal concentrations. **J Am Coll Nutr,** 1998;17:124-127.

12. Elin RJ. Assessment of magnesium status. **Clin Chem,** 1987;33:1965-1970.

Chapter 14

1.   JJ, Griffiths E, (eds). **Iron and Infection**. New York: John Wiley and Sons, 1987.

2.   Emory T. Iron and Your Health. Boca Raton, Fla: CRC Press, 1991.

3.   Colgan M, Fiedler, Colgan LA. Micronutrient status of endurance athletes affects hematology and performance. **J Appl Nutr,** 1991;43:17-30.

4.   Plowman SA, McSwegin PC. The effects of iron supplementation on female cross-country runners. **J Sports Med,** 1981;21:407-416.

5.   Hunding A, et al. Runner's anemia and iron deficiency. **Acta Med Scand**, 1981;209:315-320.

6.   Shepard RJ, Shek PN. Immunological hazards from nutritional imbalances in athletes. **Exerc Immunol Rev,** 1998;4:22-48.

7.   Nielsen P, Nachtigall D. Iron supplementation in athletes. Current recommendations. **Sports Med,** 1998;26:207-216.

8.   Vellar OD. Studies on sweat loss of nutrients. **Scand J Clin Lab Invest**, 1968;21:157-167.

9.   Williamson MR. Anemia in runners and other athletes. **Physician Sports Med**, 1981;9:73-78.

10. Ehn L, et al. Iron status in athletes involved in intense physical activity. **Med Sci Sports Exerc,** 1980;12:61-70.

11. Refsum HE, et al. Hematological changes following prolonged heavy exercise. In Jokl E, et al. (eds). **Advances In Exercise Physiology, Volume 9,** Basel:Karger;1976:91-99.

12. Colgan M, et al. Effects of multi-nutrient supplementation on athletic performance. In Katch F, (ed). **Sport Health and Nutrition**. Champaign IL:Human Kinetics;1986:59-80.

13. Selby GB, Eichner ER. Endurance swimming intravascular hemolysis and iron depletion. **Am J Med**, 1986;81:791-794.

14. Eichner ER, et al. Intravascular hemolysis in elite college rowers. **Med Sci Sports Exerc.** 1989;(Suppl):Abstract No. 466.

15. Fisher RL, et al. Gastrointestinal bleeding in competitive runners. **Digest Dis Sci,** 1986;31:1226.

16. Puhl JL, Runyan WS. Hematological variations during aerobic training of college women. **Res Quart Exer Sport,** 1980;51:533-541.

17. Jenkins RR. Free radical chemistry: relationship to exercise. **Sports Med,** 1988;5:156-170.

18. Russer WL, et al. Iron deficiency in female athletes. Med Sci Sports Exerc. 1988,20:116-121.

19. Maughan RJ ,et al. Role of micronutrients in sport and physical activity. **Br Med Bull,** 1999;55:683-690.

20. Chatard JC, et al. Anaemia and iron deficiency in athletes. Practical recommendations for treatment. **Sports Med,** 1999;27:229-240.

21. Constantini NW, et al. Iron status of highly active adolescents: evidence of depleted iron stores in gymnasts. **Int J Sports Nutr Exerc Metab,** 2000;10:62-70.

22. Faber M, Benade AJ. Mineral and vitamin intake in field athletes (discus- ,hammer-,javelin-throwers and shotputters). **Int J Sports Med,** 1991;12:324-327.

23. Beard J, Tobin B. Iron Status and exercise. **Am J Clin Nutr,** 2000;72(Suppl):594S-597S.

24. Clarkson PM, Haymes EM. Exercise and mineral status of athletes: calcium, magnesium, phosphorus, and iron. **Med Sci Sports Exerc,** 1995;27:831-843.

25. Ziegler, PJ, et al. Nutritional and physiological status of US national figure skaters. **Int J Sport Nutr,** 1999;9:345-360.

26. Ronsen O, et al. Supplement use and nutritional habits in Norwegian elite athletes. **Scand J Med Sci Sports,** 1999;9:28-35.

27. Spodaryk K. Hematological and iron related parameters in male endurance and strength-trained athletes. **Eur J Appl Physiol,** 1993;67:66.

28. Pate RR, et al. Iron status of female runners. **Int J Sports Nutr,** 1993;3:222.

Chapter 15

1. Hambidge KM, et al. Zinc. In Mertz W, (ed). **Trace Elements In Human And Animal Nutrition, Fifth Edition**. Orlando, Florida,

2. Sandstrom B, et al. Zinc absorption from composite meals. The significance of wheat extraction rate, zinc, calcium and protein content in meals based on bread. **Am J Clin Nutr,** 1980;33:739-745.

3. Briefer RR, et al. Zinc intake in the US population. **J Nutr,** 2000;130(Suppl):1367S-1373S.

4. Baer Mt, King JC. Tissue zinc levels and zinc excretion during experimental zinc depletion in young men. **Am J Clin Nutr,** 1984;39:556-570.

5. Cordova A, Navas FJ. Effect of training on zinc metabolism: changes in serum and sweat concentrations in sportsmen. **Ann Nutr Metab,** 1998;42:274-282.

6. Consolazio CE. Nutrition and performance. In Johnson RE, (ed). **Progress**

in Food and Nutrition Science Volume 7. Oxford: Pergammon Press, 1983.

7.   Hambidge M. Human zinc deficiency. **J Nutr,** 2000;130: (Suppl):1344S-1349S.

8.   King JC. Assessment of zinc status. **J Nut,** 1990;120:1474.

9.   Steen SN, McKinney S. Nutrition assessment of college wrestlers. **Physician and Sportsmed,** 1986;14:100.

10.   Bazzarre TL, et al. Incidence of poor nutritional status among triathletes, endurance athletes and controls. **Med Sci Sports Exerc,** 1986;18:S90.

11.   Couzy F, et al. Zinc metabolism in athletes: influence of training, nutrition and other factors. **Int J Sports Med,** 1990;11:263-266.

12.   Deuster PA, et al. Nutritional survey of highly trained women runners. **Am J Clin Nutr,** 1986;44:954.

13.   SJ, Jeffrey DM. Iron, zinc and copper intakes of women track team members. **Fed Proc,** 1983;42:803.

14.   Jonalagadda SS, et al. Energy and nutrient intakes of the United States Women's Artistic Gymnastics Team. **Int J Sports Nutr,** 1998;8:331-344.

15.   Ziegler PJ, et al. Nuritional and physiological status of US national figure skaters. **Int J Sports Nutr,** 1999;9:345-360.

16.   Nuviala RJ, et al. Magnesium, zinc and copper status in women involved in different sports. **Int J Sports Nutr,** 1999;9:295-309.

17.   Ames BN. Micronutrient deficiencies. A major cause of DNA damage. **Ann NY Acad Sci,** 1999;889:87-106.

18.   Lucaski HC. Magnesium, zinc and chromium nutriture and physical activity. **Am J Clin Nutr,** 2000;72(Suppl):585S-593S.

19.   Prasad AS, et al. Hypocupremia induced by zinc therapy in adults. **J Am Med Assoc,** 1978;240:2166-2168.

Chapter 16

1.   Linder MC. **Biochemistry of Copper,** New York: Plenum Press, 1991.

2.   Davis GJ, Mertz W. In Mertz W, (ed). **Trace Elements in Human and Animal Nutrition, Fifth Edition.** Orlando, FLA: Academic Press, 1987:301-364.

3.   World Health Organization. Evaluation of food additives. **WHO Technical Report No 462,** Geneva: World Health Organization, 1971.

4.   National Research Council. **Medical and Biological Effects of Environmental Pollution: Copper.** Washington, DC: National Academy of Sciences, 1977.

5.   National Research Council. **Recommended Dietary Allowances, Tenth Edition.** Washington, DC: National Academy Press, 1989.

6.   Health and Welfare Canada. **Recommended Nutrient Intakes For Canadians.** Ottawa: Department of Health and Welfare, 1983.

7.   Reeves PG. Copper. In Wolinsky I, Driscoll JA, (eds). **Sports Nutrition.** Boca Raton, FLA: CRC Press, 1997, Chapter 13.

8.   Dowdy RP, Burt J. Effect of intensive long-term training on copper and iron

nutriture in man. **Fed Proc,** 1980;39:786.

9. Mason KE. A conspectus of research on copper metabolism and requirements of man. **J Nutr,** 1979;109:1979-2066.

10. Lucaski HC. Effects of exercise training on human copper and zinc nutrition. **Adv Exp Med Biol,** 1989;258:163.

11. Turnlund JR, et al. Copper absorption and retention in young men at three levels of dietary copper using the stable isotope 65Cu. **Am J Clin Nutr,** 1989;49:870-878.

12. Van den Berg CJ, et al. Ascorbic acid feeding of rats reduces copper absorption, causing impaired copper status and depressed biliary copper excretion. **Biol Trace Elem Res,** 1994;41-47.

Chapter 17

1. Hetzel BS, Maberly GF. Iodine. In Mertz W, (ed) **Trace Elements in Human and Animal Nutrition, 5th Edition.** New York: Academic Press, 1986:139-208.

2. Nagataki S. Effect of excessive quantities of iodine. In **Handbook of Physiology III Endocrinology**, Washington, DC: American Physiological Society, 1974:329-344.

3. Pennington JAT, et al. Nutritional elements in US diets. Results of the Total Diet Study 1982 – 1986. **J Am Diet Assoc,** 1989;89:659-664.

4. Consolazio CF, et al. Comparison of nitrogen, calcium, and iodine excretion in arm and total body sweat. **Am J Clin Nutr,** 1966;18:443.

5. Mao IF, et al. The stability of iodine in human sweat. **Jpn J Physiol,** 1990;40:693-700.

6. Ziegler PJ, et al. Nutritional and physiological status of US national figure skaters. **Int J Sports Nutr,** 1999;9:45-60.

7. National Research Council. **Recommended Dietary Allowances, Tenth Edition.** Washington, DC: National Academy Press, 1989

Chapter 18

1. Mertz W, Schwartz K. Improved intravenous glucose tolerance as an early sign of dietary necrotic liver degeneration. **Arch Biochem Biophys**, 1955;58:504.

2. National Research Council. **Recommended Dietary Allowances, Tenth Edition.** Washington, DC: National Academy Press, 1989.

3. Mertz W. Effects and metabolism of glucose tolerance factors. **Nutr Rev**, 1975;33:129-135.

4. Anderson RA, et al. Dietary chromium intake, freely chosen diets, institutional diets and individual foods. **Biol Trace Elem Res,** 1992;32:117.

5. Kumpulainen JT, et al. Determination of chromium in selected United States

diets. **J Agric Food Chem**, 1979;27:490-494.

6.   Colgan M, Fiedler, Colgan LA. Micronutrient status of endurance athletes affects hematology and performance. **J Appl Nutr,** 1991;43:17-30.

7.   International Program on Chemical Safety. **Chromium. Environmental Health Criteria 61**. Geneva: World Health Organisation, 1988.

8.   Seidell K. Obesity, insulin resistance and diabetes – a worldwide epidemic. **Br J Nutr,** 2000;83:(Suppl):S5-S8.

9.   Anderson RA, et al. Chromium supplementation of human subjects: effects on glucose, insulin and lipid variables. **Metabolism,** 1983;32:894-899.

10.   Press R, et al. The effect of chromium picolinate on serum cholesterol and alipoprotein fractions in human subjects. **Western J Med,** 1990;152:41-45.

11.   Stoecker BJ. Chromium. In Brown ML (ed). **Present Knowledge in Nutrition, 6th Edition.** Washington, DC: International Life Sciences Institute, 1990:287.

12.   Anderson RA, et al. Effect of exercise (running) on serum glucose, insulin, glycogen and chromium excretion. **Diabetes,** 1982;31:212-216.

13.   Anderson RA, et al. Exercise effects of chromium excretion on trained and untrained men consuming a constant diet. **J Appl Physiol,** 1988;64:249.

14.   Campbell WW, et al. Effect of aerobic exercise on the trace minerals chromium, zinc and copper. **Sports Med**, 1987;4:9-18.

15.   Clarkson PM, Haymes EM. Trace mineral requirements for athletes. **Int J Sports Nutr,** 1994;4:104-119.

16.   Lukaski HC. Magnesium, zinc and chromium nutriture and physical activity. **Am J Clin Nutr,** 2000;72(Suppl):585S-593.S

17.   Hasten DL, et al. Effect of chromium picolinate on beginning weight training students. **Int J Sports Med,** 1992;2:343.

18.   Lefavi RG, et al. Efficacy of chromium supplementation in athletes: emphasis on anabolism. **Int J Sports Med,** 1992;2:111.

19.   Page TG, et al. Effect of chromium picolinate on growth and carcass characteristics of growing-finishing pigs. **Science,** 1991;69:403.

20.   Broadbent CL, et al. Characterization and structure by NMR and FTIR spectroscopy and molecular modeling of chromium picolinate and nicotinate complexes utilized for nutritional supplementation. **J Inorganic Biochem,** 1997;66:119-130.

21.   Anderson RA, et al. Lack of toxicity of chromium chloride and chromium picolinate in rats. **J Am Coll Nutr,**1997;16:273-279.

Chapter 19

1.   Rotruck JT, et al. Selenium. Biochemical role as a component of glutathione peroxidase. **Science,** 1973;588:179.

2.   Zachara B. Mammalian selenoproteins. **J Trace Elem Electrol Health Dis**, 1992;6:137.

3.   Laughlin MH, et al. Skeletal muscle oxidative capacity, antioxidant enzymes and exercise training. **J Appl Physiol,** 1990;68:2337.

4.   Sen CK, et al. Skeletal muscle and liver glutathione homeostasis in response to training, exercise and immobilization. **J Appl Physiol,** 1992;74:1265.

5.   Ji LL, et al. Antioxidant enzyme systems in rat liver and skeletal muscle: influences of selenium deficiency, chronic training and acute exercise. **Arch Biochem Biophys,** 1988;263:150.

6.   Keshan Disease Research Group. Epidemiological studies on the etiologic relationship of selenium and Keshan disease. **Chin Med J,** 1979;92:477-482.

7.   Colgan M. Trace elements. **Science,** 1981;214:744.

8.   National Research Council. **Recommended Dietary Allowances, Tenth Edition.** Washington, DC: National Academy Press, 1989.

9.   Duffield AJ, Thomson CD. A comparison of assessment of dietary selenium intakes in Otago, New Zealand. **Br J Nutr,** 1999;82:131-138.

10.   Levander OA. The selenium – coxsackievirus connection: chronicle of a collaboration. **J Nutr,** 2000;130(Suppl):485S-488S.

11.   Levander OA. Selenium requirements as discussed in the 1996 joint FAO/IAEA/WHO expert consultation on trace elements in human nutrition. **Biomed Environ Sci,** 1997;10:214-219.

12.   Colgan M. **Optimum Sports Nutrition.** New York, Advanced Research Press, 1993.

13.   Whanger FD, et al. Blood selenium and glutathione peroxidase activity of populations in New Zealand, Oregon and South Dakota. **FASEB,** 1988;2:2996-3002.

14.   Kryukov GV, et al. New mammalian selenocysteine-containing proteins identified with an algorithm that searches for selenocysteine insertion sequence elements. **J Biol Chem,** 1999;274:33888-33897.

15.   Bouvier N, Millart H. Relationships between selenium deficiency and 3,5,3'-triiodothyronine (T3) synthesis. **Ann Endocrinol,** 1997;58:310-315.

16.   Combs GF Jr. Chemopreventive mechanisms of selenium. **Med Klin,** 1999;94(Suppl 3):18-24.

17.   Patterson BH, Levander OA. Naturally occurring selenium compounds in cancer chemopreventive trials: a workshop summary. **Cancer Epidemiol Biomarkers Prev,** 1997;6:63-69.

18.   J, et al. Selenium deficiency, endurance exercise capacity and antioxidant status in rats. **J Appl Physiol,** 1987;63:2532.

19.   Duthie G, et al. Blood antioxidant status and lipid peroxidation following distance running. **Arch Biochem Biophys,** 1990;78:282.

Chapter 20

Manganese

1.   Hurley JS, Keen Ch. Manganese. In Mertz, (ed). **Trace Elements in Human and Animal Nutrition, 5th Edition,** New York: Academic Press, 1987:185-223.

2.   Pennington JAT, et al. Nutritional elements in US diets. Results of the Total

Diet Study 1982 – 1986. **J Am Diet Assoc,** 1989;89:659-664.

3. National Research Council. **Recommended Dietary Allowances, Tenth Edition.** Washington, DC: National Academy Press, 1989.
4. Mertz W. Use and misuse of balance studies. **J Nutr,** 1987;117:1811-1813.
5. Naslodin VV, et al. Microelements balance and correction in athletes under high muscular load. **Vopr Pitan,** 1997;4:13-15.
6. Greger JL. Dietary standards for manganese: overlap between nutritional and toxicological studies. **J Nutr,** 1998;128(2 Suppl):368S-371S.
7. Greger JL. Nutrition versus toxicology of manganese in humans: evaluation of potential biomarkers. **Neurotoxicology,** 1999;20:205-212.

Molybdenum

1. Rajagopalan KV. Molybdenum: an essential trace element in human nutrition. **Ann Rev Nutr**, 1988;8:401-427.
2. Abumrad NN, et al. Amino acid intolerance during prolonged total parenteral Nutrition reversed by molybdate therapy. **Am J Clin Nutr,** 1981;34:2551-2559.
3. Wolinsky I, Driskoll JA. **Sports Nutrition.** Boca Raton, Fla: CRC Press 1997.
4. Mills CF, Davis GK. Molybdenum. in Mertz W, (ed). **Trace Elements In Human and Animal Nutrition, 5th Edition,** New York: Academic Press, 1987:429-463.
5. Turnlund JR, et al. Molybdenum absorption and utilization in humans from soy and kale intrinsically labeled with stable isotopes of molybdenum. **Am J Clin Nutr,** 1999;69:1217-23.
6. National Research Council. **Recommended Dietary Allowances, Tenth Edition**. Washington, DC: National Academy Press, 1989.
7. Turnlund JR, et al. Molybdenum absorption, excretion, and retention studied with stable isotopes in young men at five intakes of dietary molybdenum. **Am J Clin Nutr**, 1995;62:790-796.
8. Failla ML. Consideration for determining "optimal nutrition" for copper, zinc, manganese and molybdenum. **Proc Nutr Soc,** 1999;58:497-505.

Chapter 21

Silicon

1. Carlisle EM. Silicon. In Mertz W, (ed). **Trace Elements In Humans and Animal Nutrition, 5th Edition.** New York: Academic Press, 1986:373-390.
2. Nielsen FH. Nutritional requirements for boron, silicon, vanadium, nickel, and arsenic: current knowledge and speculation. **FASAB J** 1991;5:2661-2667.
3. Uthus EO, Seaborn CD. Deliberations and evaluations of the approaches, endpoints and paradigms for dietary recommendations of the other trace ele-

ments. **J Nutr,** 1996;126(9 Suppl):2452S-2459S.

4. Pennington JA. Silicon in foods and diets. **Food Addit Contam,** 1991;8:97-118.

5. Nasolodin VV, et al. Zinc and silicon metabolism in highly trained athletes during heavy exercise. **Vopr Pitan,** 1987;Jul-Aug;4:37-39.

Boron

1. Hunt CD, Nielsen FH. Interactions between boron and cholecalciferol in the chick. In McHowell J, et al, (eds). **Trace Element Metabolism in Man and Animals Vol 4,** Canberra: Australian Academy of Science, 1981:597-600.

2. Nielsen FH. The justification for providing dietary guidance for the nutritional intake of boron. **Biol Trace Elem Res,** 1998;66:319-330.

3. Colgan M. Boron. **Nutrition and Fitness,** 1988;7:33.

4. Rainey CJ, et al. Daily boron intake from the American diet. **J Am Diet Assoc,** 1999;99:335-340.

5. Naghii MR. The significance of dietary boron, with particular reference to athletes. **Nutr Health,** 1999;13:31-37.

6. Hunt CD. Regulation of enzymatic activity: one possible role of dietary boron in higher animals and humans. **Biol Trace Elem Res,** 1998;66:205-225.

7. Neilsen FH. Possible future implications of ultrtrace elements in human health and disease. In Prasad AS,(ed). **Trace Elements In Human Health and Disease, Vol 18,** New York: Alan R Liss, 1988:277-292.

8. Hunt CD, et al. Metabolic responses of postmenopausal women to supplementary dietary boron and aluminum during usual and low magnesium intake: boron, calcium, and magnesium absorption and retention and blood mineral concentrations. **Am J Clin Nutr, 1997;65:803-813.**

9. Samman S, et al. The nutritional and metabolic effects of boron in humans and animals. **Biol Trace Elem Res,** 1998;66:227-235.

10. Meacham SL, et al. Effects of boron supplementation on bone mineral density and dietary, blood, and urinary, calcium, phosphorus, magnesium, and boron in female athletes. **Environ Health Perspect,** 1994;102 Suppl 7:79-82.

11. Naghii MR. The significance of dietary boron, with particular reference to athletes. **Nutr Health,** 1999;13:31-37.

Chapter 22

Vanadium

1. Neilsen FH. Possible future implications of ultratrace elements in human health and disease. In Prasad AS,(ed). **Trace Elements In Human Health and Disease, Vol 18,** New York: Alan R Liss, 1988:277-292.

2. Heyliger CE, et al. Effect of vanadate on elevated blood glucose and depressed cardiac performance of diabetic rats. **Science,** 1985;227:757-759.

3.   Poucheret P, et al. Vanadium and diabetes. **Mol Cell Biochem,** 1998;188:73-80.

4.   Ramandham S, et al. Oral vanadate in treatment of diabetes mellitus in rats. **Amer J Physiol,** 1989;257:H904-H911.

5.   Cam MC, et al. Long-term effectiveness of oral vanadyl sulphate in streptozotocin-diabetic rats. **Diabetologia,** 1993;36:218-24.

6.   Domingo JL. Improvement of glucose homeostasis by oral vanadyl or vanadate treatment in diabetic rats is accompanied by negative side effects. **Pharm Toxic,** 1991;68:249-253.

7.   Barceloux DG. Vanadium. **J Toxicol Clin Toxicol,** 1999;37:265-278.

Arsenic

1.   Neilsen FH. Possible future implications of ultratrace elements in human health and disease. In Prasad AS,(ed). **Trace Elements In Human Health and Disease, Vol 18,** New York: Alan R Liss, 1988:277-292.

2.   Tao SS, Bolger PM. Dietary arsenic intakes in the United States: FDA Total Diet Study, September 1991-December 1996.   **Food Addit Contam,** 1999;16:465-472.

3.   Schoof RA, et al. A market basket survey of inorganic arsenic in food. **Food Chem Toxicol,** 1999;37:839-846.

Chapter 23

1.   Dean HT et al. Domestic water and dental caries. **Public Health Rep,** 1942;57:1155-1179.

2.   Council on Dental Therapeutics, **Accepted Dental Therapeutics, 39th Edition.** Chicago IL: American Dental Association, 1982:344-368.

3.   Krishnamachari KA. Fluorine. In Mertz W, (ed). **Trace Elements in Human and Animal Nutrition.** New York: Academic Press, 1987:365-415.

4.   US National Research Council. Fluorides. **Report of the Committee on Biologic Effects of Atmospheric Pollutants.** Washington, DC: National Academy of Sciences, 1971.

5.   Dabeka RW, McKenzie AD. Survey of lead, cadmium, fluoride, nickel, and cobalt in food composites and estimation of dietary intakes of these elements by Canadians in 1986-1988. **J AOAC Int,** 1995;78:897-909.

6.   Full CA, Parkins FM. Effect of cooking vessel composition on fluoride. **J Dent Res,** 1975;54:192.

7.   Walters CB, et al. Dietary intake of fluoride in the United Kingdom and fluoride content of some foodstuffs. **J Sci Food Agric,** 1983;34:523-528.

Chapter 24

1. National Research Council. **Recommended Dietary Allowances, Tenth Edition**. Washington, DC: National Academy Press, 1989.
2. Neve J. The nutritional importance and pharmacologic effects of cobalt and vitamin B12 in man. **J Pharm Belg**, 1991;46:271-280.
3. Neilsen FH. Possible future implications of ultratrace elements in human health and disease. In Prasad AS,(ed). **Trace Elements In Human Health and Disease, Vol 18,** New York: Alan R Liss, 1988:277-292.
4. Pekclharing HL, et al. Iron, copper and zinc status in rats fed on diets containing various concentrations of tin. Br J Nutr, 1994;71:103-109.
5. Beynen AC, et al. High intakes of tin lower iron status in rats. **Biol Trace Elem Res,** 1992;35:85-88.
6. Rader JI. Anti-nutritive effects of dietary tin. **Adv Exp Med Biol,** 1991;289:509-524.
7. Dabeka RW, McKenzie AD. Survey of lead, cadmium, fluoride, nickel, and cobalt in food composites and estimation of dietary intakes of these elements by Canadians in 1986-1988. **J AOAC Int,** 1995;78:897-909.
8. Biego GH, et al. Daily intake of essential minerals and metallic micropollutants from foods in France. **Sci Total Environ,** 1998;217:27-36.
9. Schauss AG. Nephrotoxicity in humans by the ultratrace element germanium. **Ren Fail,** 1991;13:1-4.

Chapter 25

1. National Research Council. **Recommended Dietary Allowances, 10th Ed**. Washington, DC: National Academy Press, 1989.
2. Colgan M. **Optimum Sports Nutrition**. New York, NY: Advanced Research Press, 1993.
3. Colgan M. **The New Nutrition**. Vancouver, BC: Apple Publishing, 1995.
4. Colgan M. **Hormonal Health**. Vancouver, BC: Apple Publishing, 1996.
5. Colgan M. **Your Personal Vitamin Profile**. New York, NY: William Morrow, 1983.
6. Oakley GP. Eat right and take a multivitamin. **New Engl J Med**, 1998;338:1060-1061.

Chapter 26

1. Goodman DS. Vitamin A and retinoids in health and disease. **New Engl J Med**, 1984;310:1023-1031.
2. Novotny JA, et al. Compartmental analysis of the dynamics of beta-carotene metabolism in an adult volunteer. **J Lipid Res**, 1995;36:1825.
3. Stacewitz-Sapuntzakis M in Wolinsky I, Driscoll JA. (eds). **Sports Nutrition**.

Boca Raton, Florida: CRC Press, 1997:101-118.

4. Kobylinski Z, et al. Effect of exercise on vitamin A utilization by rat organism. **Rocz Panstuf Zoki Hig**, 1990;41:247.
5. Sauerlich HE, et al. **Laboratory Tests For The Assessment of Nutritional Status**, Cleveland OH; CRC Press, 1976.
6. Kanini JJ, et al. Preclinical and clinical toxicity of selected retinoids. In Sporn MB, et al. (eds). **The Retinoids Volume 2**. New York: Academic Press, 1984; 288.

Chapter 27

1. Shils ME, Olsen JA, (eds). **Modern Nutrition in Health and Disease**. Philadelphia, MA: Lea and Febiger, 1994.
2. Harris RS, Karmas E, (eds). **Nutritional Evaluation of Food Processing**. Westport, CT: AVI Publishing, 1975.
3. Hickson JK, et al. Nutritional intake from food sources of soccer athletes during two stages of training. **Nutr Rep Int**, 1986;34:85.
4. Giulland JC, et al. Vitamin status of young athletes including the effects of supplementation. **Med Sci Sports Exer**, 1989;21:441.
5. Sauerlich HE, et al. **Laboratory Tests For The Assessment of Nutritional Status**. Cleveland, OH: CRC Press, 1976.
6. National Research Council. **Recommended Dietary Allowances, 10ᵗʰ Ed**. Washington, DC: National Academy Press, 1989.

Chapter 28

1. Belko AZ, et al. Effects of exercise on riboflavin requirements of young women. **Am J Clin Nutr**, 1983;37:509-517.
2. Harris RS, Karmas E, (eds). **Modern Nutrition In Health and Disease**. Philadelphia, MA: Lea and Febiger, 1994.
3. Haralambie G. Vitamin B_{12} status in athletes and the influence of riboflavin administration on neuromuscular irritability. **Nutr Metab**, 1976;20:1.
4. Short SH. Surveys of dietary intake and nutrition knowledge of athletes and their coaches. In Wolinsky I, Hickson JF, (eds). **Nutrition In Exercise and Sport**. Boca Raton, FL: CRC Press, 1994.
5. Campbell TC, et al. Questioning riboflavin recommendations on the basis of a survey in China. **Am J Clin Nutr**, 1990;51:436.
6. Lewis D. Riboflavin and niacin. In Wolisnky I, Driskoll JA. **Sports Nutrition**. Boca Raton, FL: CRC Press, 1997:57-73.
7. Manore MM. Effect of physical activity in humans on thiamin, riboflavin and vitamin B_6 requirements. **Am J Clin Nutr**. 2000;72;Suppl:5988-6065.
8. McCormick DB. Riboflavin. In Shils ME, Young VR. **Modern Nutrition In Health and Disease**. Philadelphia, MA: Lea and Febiger, 1988:362-369.

Chapter 29

1. Swendseid ME, Jacob RA. Niacin. In Shils ME, et al, (eds). **Modern Nutrition in Health and Disease**. Malvern, PA: Lea and Febiger, 1994:376.
2. Keith RE. Vitamins and physical activity. In Wolinsky I, Hickson FJ, (eds). **Nutrition In Exercise And Sport**. Boca Raton, FL: CRC Press, 1994:159.
3. Carlson LA, et al. Effect of nicotinic acid on the turnover rate and oxidation of the free fatty acids of plasma in man during exercise. **Metab Clin Exp**, 1963;12:837.

Chapter 30

1. Huang YC, et al. Vitamin B_6 requirement and status of young women fed a high protein diet with various levels of vitamin B_6. **Am J Clin Nutr**, 1998;67:208-220.
2. Colgan M, Fiedler MS, Colgan LA. Micronutrient use of endurance athletes affects hematology and performance. **J Appl Nutr**, 1991;43:16-30.
3. Rozitzki L, et al. Assessment of vitamin B_6 status of strength and speed power athletes. **J Am Coll Nutr**, 1994;13:87-94.
4. Steen SN, et al. Dietary intakes of female collegiate heavyweight rowers. **Int J Sports Med**, 1995;5:225-231.
5. Giulland JC, et al. Vitamin status of young athletes including the effects of supplementation. **Med Sci Sports Exer**, 1989;21:441.
6. Rozitzki L, et al. Acute changes in vitamin B_6 status in endurance athletes before and after a marathon. **Int J Sports Med**, 1994;4:154-165.
7. Powers HJ. Current knowledge concerning optimal nutritional status of riboflavin, niacin and pyridoxine. **Prac Nutr Soc**, 1999;58:435-440.
8. Maxwell SR, et al. Changes in plasma antioxidant status during eccentric exercise and the effect of vitamin supplementation. **Free Rad Res Commun**, 1993;19:191.
9. Ji L. Oxidative stress during exercise: implications of antioxidant nutrients. **Free Rad Biol Med**, 1995;18:1079.

Chapter 31

1. Johnson RK, Kennedy E. The 2000 dietary guidelines for Americans: what are the changes and why were they made? **J Am Diet Assoc**, 2000;100:769-774.
2. Dwyer J. Old wine in new bottles? – The RDA and the DRI. **Nutrition**, 2000;16:488-492.
3. National Research Council. **Recommended Dietary Allowances, 10th Ed**. Washington, DC: National Academy Press, 1989.
4. Ames B. Micronutrient deficiencies: A major cause of DNA damage. **Ann**

NY Acad Sci, 1999;889:87-106.

5. Ziegler PJ, et al. Nutritional and physiological status of US national figure skaters. **Int J Sport Nutr**, 1999;345-360.

6. Barry A, et al. A nutritional study of Irish athletes. **Brit J Sports Med**, 1981;15:99-106.

7. Singh A, et al. Dietary intake and biochemical profiles of nutritional status of ultra-marathoners. **Med Sci Sports Exer**, 1993;25:328-332.

8. Schilling RF. Intrinsic factor studies II. The effect of gastric juice on the urinary excretions of radioactivity after the oral administration of radioactive B_{12}. **J Lab Clin Med**, 1953;42:860-865.

9. Keith RE. In Hickson JF, Wolinsky I, (eds). **Nutrition in Exercise and Sport**. Boca Raton, FL: CRC Press, 1989, 234-249.

Chapter 32

1. Colgan M. **Beat Arthritis**. Vancouver: Apple Publishing, 2000.

2. Colgan M. **Your Personal Vitamin Profile**. New York, NY: William Morrow, 1983.

3. National Research Council. **Recommended Dietary Allowances, 10th Ed**. Washington, DC: National Academy Press, 1989.

4. de Bree A, et al. Folate intake in Europe, recommended, actual and desired intake. **Eur J Clin Nutr**, 1997;51:643-660.

5. Bates CJ, et al. Plasma total homocysteine in a representative sample of 972 British men and women aged 65 and over. **Eur J Clin Nutr**. 1997;51:691-697.

6. Ward M, et al. Plasma homocysteine, a risk factor for cardiovascular disease is lowered by physiological doses of folic acid. **Quar J Med**, 1997;90:519-524.

7. Centers for Disease Control. Recommendations for the use of folic acid to reduce the number of cases of spina bifida and other neural defects. **Morb Mortal Wkly Rep**, 1992;41:1-7.

8. Ames BN. A major cause of DNA damage. **Ann NY Acad Sci**, 1999;889:87-106.

9. Lucock M. Folic acid in nutritional biochemistry, molecular biology, and role in disease processes. **Mol Genet Metab**, 2000;71:121-138.

10. Lucock M, Dasokalakis I. New Perspective on folate status: a differential role for the vitamin in cardiovascular disease, birth defects and other conditions. **Brit J Biomed Sci**, 2000;57:254-260.11.

12. Barry A, et al. A nutritional study of Irish athletes. **Brit J Sports Med**, 1981;15:99-101.

13. Singh A, et al. Dietary intakes and biochemical profiles of nutritional status of ultramarathoners. **Med Sci Sports Exer**, 1993;25:328-334.

Chapter 33

1.   Dakshinamarti K, Bhagavan HN, (eds). **Biotin in Human Nutrition**. New York: New York Academy of Sciences, 1985.
2.   National Research Council. **Recommended Dietary Allowances, 10ᵗʰ Ed**. Washington, DC: National Academy Press, 1989.
3.   Baugh CM, et al. Human biotin deficiency. **Am J Clin Nutr**, 1968;21:173-182.
4.   Singh A, et al. Vitamin and mineral status in physically active men: effects of a high potency supplement. **Am J Clin Nutr**, 1992;55:1-6.
5.   Hentz NG, Bachas LG. Fluorophore-linked assays for high performance liquid chromatography post-calcium reduction detection of biotin and biocytin. **Methods Enzymol**, 1997;279:275-286.

Chapter 34

1.   National Research Council. **Recommended Dietary Allowances, 10ᵗʰ Ed**. Washington, DC: National Academy Press, 1989.
2.   Combs GF. **Pantothenic Acid. In The Vitamins: Fundamental Aspects in Nutrition and Health**. San Diego, CA: Academic Press, 1992:345.
3.   Rozitzki L, et al. Pantothenic acid levels in blood of athletes at rest and after aerobic exercise. **Z Ernahrungswiss**, 1993;32:282-288.
4.   Litoff D, et al. Effects of pantothenic acid on human exercise. **Med Sci Sports Exerc**, 1985;17:287 (abstract).
5.   Nice C, et al. The effects of pantothenic acid on human exercise capacity. **J Sports Med**, 1984;24:26-29.

Chapter 35

1.   Basu TK, Schorah CJ. **Vitamin C In Health and Disease**, Westport, CT: AVI Publishing, 1982.
2.   Colgan M. **Your Personal Vitamin Profile**. New York, NY: William Morrow, 1983.
3.   Machlin LI, (ed). **Handbook of Vitamins, Second Edition**. New York, NY: Marcel Dekker, 1991.
4.   Colgan M. **Optimum Sports Nutrition**. New York, NY: Advanced Research Press, 1993.
5.   Keith RE. Ascorbic acid. In Wolinsky I, Driskell JA. (eds) **Sports Nutrition, Vitamins And Trace Elements**. Boca Raton, FL: CRC Press, 1997:29-45.
6.   Keith RE, Merrill E. The effects of vitamin C on maximum grip strength and muscular endurance. **J Sports Med Phys Fitness**, 1983;23:253-258.
7.   Keren B, Epstein Y. Effect of high dosage vitamin C on aerobic and anaerobic capacity. **J Sports Med Phys Fitness**, 1980;20:145-149.

8.   Howald H, et al. Ascorbic acid and athletic performance. **Ann NY Acad Sci**, 1976;258:458.
9.   Balakrishnan SD, Anuradha CV. Exercise depletion of antioxidants and antioxidant manipulation, **Cell Biochem Funct**, 1998;16:269-275.
10. Sanchez-Quesada JL, et al. Ascorbic acid inhibits the increase in low density lipoprotein LDL susceptibility to oxidation and the proportion of electronegative LDL induced by intense aerobic exercise. **Coron Art Dis**, 1998;9:249-255.
11. Vasankari T, et al. Effects of ascorbic acid and carbohydrate ingestion on exercise induced oxidative stress. **J Sports Med Phys Fitness**, 1998;38:281-285.
12. Clarkson PM, Thompson HS. **Am J Clin Nutr**, 2000;72: (Suppl): 637S-646S.
13. Schroder H, et al. Nutrition, antioxidant status and oxidative stress in professional basketball players: effects of a three compound antioxidant supplement. **Int J Sports Med**, 2000;21:146-150.
14. Mackinnon LT. Chronic exercise training effects on immune function. **Med Sci Sports Exer**, 2000;32;(Suppl):S369-S376.
15. Peters, EM. Vitamin C supplementation reduces the incidence of post-race symptoms of upper-respiratory tract infection in ultramarathon runners. **Am J Clin Nutr**, 1993;57:170.
16. Cohen HA, et al. Blocking effect of vitamin C in exercise induced asthma. **Arch Pediatr Adolesc**, 1997;151:367-370.
17. Block G, et al. Bodyweight and prior depletion affect plasma ascorbate levels attained on identical vitamin C intake. **J Am Col Nutr**, 1999;18:628-637.

Chapter 36

1.   DeLuca HF. New concepts of vitamin D functions. **Ann NY Acad Sci**, 1993;669:59-68.
2.   DeLuca HF. Vitamin D. In Goodhart R, Shilo ME, (eds). **Modern Nutrition In Health and Disease**. Philadelphia, MA: Lea and Febiger, 1980:Chapter 6.
3.   Klansen T, et al. Plasma levels of parathyroid hormone, vitamin D, calcitomin and calcium in association with endurance exercise. **Calcif Tissue Res**, 1993:52:205.
4.   National Research Council. **Recommended Dietary Allowances, 10ᵗʰ Ed**. Washington, DC: National Academy Press, 1989.

Chapter 37

1.   Meydani M. Vitamin E. **Lancet**, 1995;345:170
2.   Powers SK, Lennon SL. Analysis of cellular responses to free radicals: Focus on exercise and skeletal muscle. **Prac Nutr Soc**, 1999;58:1025-1033.

3. Neville HE, et al. Ultrastructural and histochemical abnormalities of skeletal muscle in patients with chronic vitamin E deficiency. **Neurology**, 1983;33:483-487.
4. Leonard PJ, Losowsky MS. Effect of alpha-tocopherol administration on red cell survival in vitamin E deficient human subjects. **Am J Clin Nutr**, 1971;24:388-393.
5. National Research Council. **Recommended Dietary Allowances, 10th Ed**. Washington, DC: National Academy Press, 1989:103.
6. Evans WJ. Vitamin C, vitamin E and exercise. **Am J Clin Nutr**, 2000;72(Suppl): 647S-652S.
7. Vasankari TJ, et al. Increased serum and low density lipoprotein antioxidant potential after antioxidant supplementation in endurance athletes. **Am J Clin Nutr**, 1997;65:1052-1056.
8. Murphy SP, et al. Vitamin E intake and sources in the United States. **Am J Clin Nutr**, 1990;52:361-366.
9. National Research Council. **Recommended Dietary Allowances, 10th Ed**. Washington, DC: National Academy Press, 1989.
10. Traber MG, et al. Absorption and transport of deuterium substituted 2'R.4'R.8'R-alpha-tocopherol in human lipoproteins. **Lipids**, 1988;23:791-797.
11. Farrell PM, et al. Evaluation of vitamin E deficiency in children with lung disease. **Ann NY Acad Sci**, 1982;393:96-108.
12. Bendich A, Machlin LJ. Safety of oral intake of vitamin E. **Am J Clin Nutr**, 1988;48:612-619.

Chapter 38

1. Bender DA. Vitamin K. In Bender DA, (ed). **Nutritional Biochemistry of the Vitamins**. London: Cambridge University Press; 1992:Chapter 5.
2. National Research Council. **Recommended Dietary Allowances, 10th Ed**. Washington, DC: National Academy Press, 1989.
3. Olson JA. Recommended dietary intakes (RDI) of vitamin K in humans. **Am J Clin Nutr**, 1987;45:687-692.
4. Puckett R, Offringa M. Prophylactic vitamin K for vitamin K deficiency bleeding in neonates (Cochrane Review). **Cochrane Database Syst Rev**, 2000;4:CD002776.
5. Hobart JA, Smucker DR. The female athlete triad. **Am Fam Physician**, 2000;61:3357-3367.
6. American Academy of Pediatrics. Committee on Sports Medicine and Fitness. Medical concerns of the female athlete. **Pediatrics**, 2000;106:610-613.
7. Warren MP; Stiehl AL. Exercise and female adolescents: effects on the reproductive and skeletal systems. **J Am Med Women's Assoc**. 1999;54:115-120,138.
8. Pettersson U, et al. Low bone mass density at multiple skeletal sites, includ-

ing the appendicular skeleton in amenorrheic runners. **Calcif Tissue Int**, 1999;64:117-125.

9.   Callahan LR. Stress fractures in women. **Clin Sports Med**, 2000;19:303-314.

10.   Beckvid Henriksson G, et al. Women endurance runners with menstrual dysfunction have prolonged interruption of training due to injury. **Gynecol Obstet Invest**, 2000;49:41-46.

11.   Keen AD, Drinkwater BL. Irreversible bone loss in former amenorrheic athletes. (editorial) **Osteporos Int**, 1997;7:311-315.

12.   Gibson JH, et al. Treatment of reduced bone mineral density in athletic amenorrhea: a pilot study. **Osteoporos Int**, 1999;10:284-289.

13.   Cracium AM, et al. Improved bone metabolism in female elite athletes after vitamin K supplementation. **Int J Sports Med**, 1998;19:479-484.

Chapter 40

1.   Penn D, et al. Carnitine concentrations in the milk of different species and infant formulas. **Biol Neonate**, 1987;52:70-79.

2.   Taglialagela G, et al. Acetyl-L-carnitine enhances the response of Pc12 cells to nerve growth factor. **Brain Res Dev Brain Res**, 1991;59:221-230.

3.   Bossini G, Carpi C. Effect of acetyl-L-carnitine on conditioned reflex learning rate and retention in laboratory animals. **Drugs Exp Clin Res**, 1986;12:911-916.

4.   Ramacci MT, et al. Effect of long-term treatment with acetyl-L-carnitine on structural changes of aging rat brains. **Drugs Exp Clin Res,** 1988;14:593-601.·

5.   Germia E. Antioxidant actions of acetyl-L-carnitine: In vitro study. **Med Sci Res**, 1988;16:699-700.

6.   Dowson JH, et al. The morphology of lipopigment in rat parkirge neurons after chronic acetyl-L-carnitine administration. **Bid Psych Morphon**, 1992;32:179-182.

7.   Malone H, et al. Altered neuro-exitability in experimental diabetic neuropathy effect of acetyl-L-carnitine. **Int J Clin Pharmacol**, 1992;12:237-241.

8.   Cunti D, et al. Effect of aging and acetyl-L-carnitine on energetic and cholinergic metabolism in rat brain regions. **Mesch Aging Devt,** 1989;47:39-45.

9.   White HL, Scates PW. Acetyl-L-carnitine as a precursor of acetylcholine. **Neurochem Res**, 1990;15:597-601.

10.   Pettigrew JW, et al. Chemical and neurochemical effects of acetyl-L-carnitine in Alzheimer's disease. **Neurobiol Aging,** 1995;16:1-4.

11.   Cucinotti D, et al. Multicenter clinical placebo-controlled study with acetyl-L-carnitine in the treatment of mildly demented elderly patients. **Drug Dev Res,** 1988;14:213-216.

12.   Lino A, et al. Psycho-functional changes in attention and learning under the action of acetyl-L-carnitine in 17 young subjects. **Clin Ther**, 1992;140:569-543.

13. Sershon H, et al. Effect of acetyl-L-carnitine on the dopaminergic systems in aging animals. **J Neurosci**, 1991;30:555-559.
14. Napoleone P, et al. Age dependent nerve cell loss in the brain of Sprogue-Dawley rats: Effect of long-term acetyl-L-carnitine treatment. **Arch Gerontal Geriat**, 1990;10:173-185.

Chapter 41

1. Sun AY, Sun GH. Neurochemical aspects of the membrane hypothesis of aging. **Interdiscp Topics Gerontol**, 1979;15:34-53.
2. Schroeder F. Role of lipid membrane asymmetry in aging. **Neurobiol Aging**, 1984;5:323-333.
3. Nolan KA, Blass JP. Preventing cognitive decline. **Clin Geriat**, 1992:8:19-34.
4. Bartus RT, et al. The cholinergic hypothesis of geriatric memory dysfunction. **Science**, 1982;217:408-417.
5. Ginidin J. The effect of plant phosphatidylserine on age associated memory impairment and mood in the functioning elderly. **Gerontologist**, 1993;33:Abstract.
6. Double-blind crossover study of phosphatidylserine vs placebo in patients with early dementia of the Alzheimer's type. **Eur Neuropsychopharmacol**, 1992;2:149-155.
7. Crook TH, et al. Effects of phosphatidylserine in age associated memory impairment. **Neurol**, 1991;41:644-649.
8. Heiss WD, et al. Long-term effects of phosphatidylserine, pyritinol and cognitive training in Alzheimer's disease. **Dementia**, 1994;5:88-98.
9. Ammasari-Teule M, et al. Chronic administration of phosphatidylserine during ontogeny enhances subject environment interactions and radial maze performance in C57/B46 mice. **Physiol Behav**, 1990;47:755-760.

Chapter 42

1. Reiter, RJ, **Trends in Endocrinology and Metabolism,** 1991;1:13-19.
2. Pierpaoli W, et al (eds). **The Aging Clock**. New York: New York Academy of Sciences, 1994.
3. Reiter, RJ, et al. A review of the evidence supporting melatonin's role as an antioxidant. **J Pineal Res,** 1995;18:1-11.
4. Maestroni GJ, et al. Pineal melatonin: Its fundamental immunoregulatory role in aging and cancer. **Ann NY Acad Sci**, 1988;521:140-148.
5. Dawson D, Encel N. Melatonin and sleep in humans. **J Pineal Res**, 1993;15:1-12.
6. Valcavi R, et al. Melatonin stimulates growth hormone secretion through pathways other than the growth hormone releasing hormone. **Clin**

Endocrinol, 1993;39:193-199.
7. Dakshinamurti K, et al. Neurobiology of pyridoxine. **Ann NY Acad Sci,** 1990;585:128-144.
8. Colgan M. **Optimum Sports Nutrition**. New York: Advanced Research Press, 1993.
9. Colgan M. **The New Nutrition: Medicine for the Millennium.** Vancouver: Apple Publishing, 1994.

Chapter 43

1. McCully KS. Homocysteine, Folate, Vitamin B12 and cardiovascular disease. **JAMA**, 1998;279:392-393.
2. Rimm EB, et al. Folate and vitamin B12 from diet and supplements in relation to risk of coronary heart disease in women. **JAMA**, 1998;279:359-365.
3. Regland B, et al. Increased concentrations of homocysteine in the cerebrospinal fluid in patients with fibromyalgia and chronic fatigue syndrome. **Scand J Rheumatol,** 1997;26:301-307.
4. Parnetti L, et al. Role of homocysteine in age related vascular and non-vascular disorders. **Aging (Milan),** 1997;4:241-257.
5. Fava M, et al. Folate, vitamin B12 and homocysteine in major depressive disorders. **Am J Psychiat**, 1997;154:426-428.
6. Roubenoff R, et al. Abnormal homocysteine metabolism in rheumatoid arthritis. **Arth Rheum,** 1997;40:718-722.
7. Joosten E, et al. Is metabolic evidence for vitamin B12 and folate deficiency more frequent in elderly patients with Alzheimer's. **J Geront,** 1997;52:M76-79.
8. Bottiglieri T, et al. Folate, vitamin B12 and neuropozehiatine disorders. **Nutr Rev**, 1996;54:382-390.
9. Graham IM, et al. Plasma homocysteine as a risk factor for vascular disease. The European Concerted Action Project. **JAMA**, 1997;277:1775-1781.
10. de Bree A, et al. Folate intake in Europe: recommended, actual and desired intake. Department of Human Nutrition, Wageningen Agricultural University, the Netherlands.
11. **US RDA Handbook, 10th Edition**. Washington, DC: National Academy Press, 1989.
12. Bates CJ, et al. Plasma total homocysteine in a representative sample of 972 British men and women aged 65 and over. **Eur J Clin Nutr,** 1997;10:691-697.
13. Evers S, et al. Features, symptoms and neurophysiological findings in stroke associated with hyperhomocystinemia. **Arch Neurol,** 1997;10:1276-1282.
14. Ward M, et al. Plasma homocysteine, a risk factor for cardiovascular disease,

is lowered by physiological doses of folic acid. **Quar J Med,** 1997;90:519-524.

15. Malinow M, et al. Reduction of plasma homocyst (e) ine levels by breakfast cereal fortified with folic acid in patients with coronary heart disease. **N Engl J Med,** 1998;338(15):1009-1015.
16. Moghadasian MH, et al. Homocysteine and coronary evidence and genetic and metabolic background. **Arch Int Med,** 1997;157:2299-2308.
17. Stabler SP, et al. Vitamin B12 deficiency in the elderly: current dilemmas. **Am J Clin Nutr,** 1997;66:741-749.
18. Loehrer FM, et al. Influence of oral S-adenosylmethionine on plasma 5-methyltetrahydrofolate, S-adenosylhomocysteine, homocysteine and methionine in healthy humans. **J Pharmacol Exp Ther,** 1997;282:845-850.

Chapter 44

1. Colgan M. **The Power Program.** San Diego: CI Publications, 1991.
2. Soderlund K, Hultman E. ATP and phosphcreatine changes in single human muscle fibers after intense electrical stimulation. **Amer J Physiol,** 1991: 261:E737-E741.
3. Harris R, et al. Elevation of creatine in resting and exercise muscles of normal subjects by creatine supplementation. **Clin Sci,** 1992:83:367-374.
4. Greenhaff P. Creatine and its application as an ergogenic aid. **Int J Sports Nutr,** 1995:5:S100-S110.
5. Balsom PD, et al. Skeletal muscle metabolism during short duration, high intensity exercise: influence of creatine supplementation. **Acta Physiol Scand,** 1995:154:303-310
6. Balsom P, et al. Creatine in humans with special reference to creatine supplementation. Sports Med, 1994:18:268-280.
7. C, et al. The effect of creatine monohydrate ingestion on anaerobic power indices, muscular strength and body composition. **Acta Physiol Scand,** 1995: 153:207-209.
8. Balsom P, et al. Creatine supplementation and dynamic high-intensity intermittent exercise. **Scand J Med Sci Sports,** 1993;3:143-149.
9. Sahelian R, Tuttle D. **Creatine: Nature's Muscle Builder.** New York: Avery Publishing, 1997.
   Bosco C, et al. Effect of oral creatine supplementation on jumping and running performance. **Int J Sports Med,** 1997;18:369-72.
9. Vandenberghe K, et al. Long-term creatine intake is beneficial to muscle performance during resistance training. **J Appl Physiol,** 1997;83:2055-63.
10. Prevost MC, et al. Creatine supplementation enhances intermittent work performance. **Res Q Exerc Sport,** 1997;68:233-40.
11. Engelhardt R, et al. Creatine supplementation in endurance sports. **Med Sci Sports Exerc,** 1998;30:1123-1129.
12. Colgan m. **Hormonal Health,** Vancouver: Apple Publishing 1994
13. jrstout@creighton.edu, e-mail to Colgan Institute 7 January 1999.

Chapter 45

1. Colgan M. **Optimum Sports Nutrition**. New York: Advanced Research Press, 1993.
2. Steiner J. Absorption, distribution and excretion of radioactivity after a single intravenous or oral administration of glucosamine to the rat. **Pharmatherapeutics**, 1984;3:538-550.
3. Setnikar J. Pharmacokinetics of glucosamine in the dog and man. **Arneimittelforschung**, 1991;36:729-736.
4. Vaz AL. Double-blind evaluation of the relative efficacy of glucosamine sulfate in the management of osteoarthritis of the knee. **Curr Med Res Opin,** 1982;8:145-149.
5. Bohmen D, et al (eds). Treatment of chondropathia patellae in young athletes with glucosamine sulfate. **Current Topics In Sports Medicine,** Vienna: Urban and Schwarzenberg, 1984.
6. Andermann G, Dietz M. The influence of the route of administration on the bioavailability of an endogenous macromolecule, chondroitin sulfate (CSA). **Eur J Drug Metab Pharm Pharmacokinet**, 1982;7:11-16.
7. Pescador R, Madonna M. Pharmokinetics of fluorescin-labeled glycosamino-glycans and of their lipoprotein lipase-inducing activity in the rat. **Arzneim-Forsch Drug Res**, 1982;32:819-824.
8. Clevidence BA, et al. Pharmacokinetics of catalytically tritiated gly-cosaminoglycans in the rat. **Arzneim-Forsh**, 1983;33(2):228-230.
9. Baici A, et al. Analysis of glycosaminoglycans in human serum after oral administration of chondroitin sulfate. **Rheumatol Int**, 1992;12:81-88.
10. Morreal P, et al. Comparison of the anti-inflammatory efficacy of chondroitin sulfate and diclofenac sodium in patients with knee osteoarthritis. **J Rheumatol**, 1996;23:1385-1391.
11. Conte A, et al. Biochemical and pharmacokinetic aspects of oral treatment with chondroitin sulfate. **Arzneim-Forsh**, 1995, Aug;45(8):918-925.
12. Silvestro L, et al. Human pharmacokinetics of glycosaminoglycans using deuterium-labeled and unlabeled substances: evidence for oral absorption. **Semin Thromb Hemost,** 1994;20:281-292.
13. Gustafson S. The influence of sulfated polysaccharides on the circulating levels of hyaluronan. **Glycobiology**, 1997;7(8):1209-1214.
14. Hutadilok N, et al. **Ther Res,** 1988;44:845.
15. Bassleer C, et al. Int J Tassne React, 1992;14:231.
16. Barcelo HA, et al. Effect of S-adenosylmethionine on experimental osteoarthritis in rabbits. **Am J Med,** 1987;83:55-59.
17. Stramentinoli G. Pharmacological aspects of S-adenosylmethionine. **Am J Med,** 1987;83:35-42.
18. di Padova C. S-adenosylmethionine in the treatment of osteoarthritis. Review of the clinical studies. **Am J Med,** 1987;83:60-65.
19. Gutierres S, et al. **Brit J Rheumatol**, 1997;36:27-31.

20. Colgan M. **Essential Fats.** Vancouver: Apple Publishing, 1998.
21. Muller-Fassbender H. Double-blind clinical trial of S-adenosylmethionine versus ibuprofen in the treatment of osteoarthritis. **Am J Med,** 1987;83:81-83.
22. Caruso I, Pietrogrande V. Italian double-blind multi-center study comparing S-adenosylmethionine, naproxsyn and placebo in the treatment of degenerative joint disease. **Am J Med,** 1987;38:66-71.
23. Maccagno A, et al. Double-blind controlled clinical trial of oral S-adenosyl-methionine versus peroxicam in knee osteoarthritis. **Am J Med,** 1987;83:72-77.
24. Konig B. A long-term (two years) clinical trial with S-adenosylmethionine for the treatment of osteoarthritis. **Am J Med,** 1987;83:89-94.

Chapter 46

1. Messina MJ, et al. Soy intake and cancer: a review of the in vitro and in vivo data. **Nutr Cancer,** 1994;21:113-131.
2. Messina MJ, et al(eds). Second International Symposium on the Role of Soy in Preventing and Treating Chronic Discases. Brussels, Belgium; 19 Sept. 1996:36.
3. Colgan M. **The New Nutrition.** Vancouver: Apple Publishing, 1995.
4. American Heart Association, Heart and Stroke Facts, 1996. **Statistical Supplement. AHA,** 1996.
5. National Cholesterol Education Program Expert Panel. **NIH Publication No. 91-2732,** 1991.
6. Wolfe BM, et al. Hypolipidemic effect of substituting soybean protein isolate for all meat and dairy products in the diets of hypercholesterolemic men, **Nutr Rep Int,** 1981;24:1187-1198.
7. Potter SM, et al. Depression of plasma cholesterol in men by consumption of baked products containing soy protein. **Am J Clin Nutr,** 1993;58:501-506.
8. Wang MF, et al. Antihypercholesterolemic effect of undigested fraction of soybean protein in young female volunteers. **J Nutr Sci Vitaminol,** 1995;41:187-195.
9. Kritchevsky D. Dietary protein and experimental atherosclerosis. **Ann NY Acad Sci,** 1993;676:180-187.
10. Kurowska EM, Carroll KK. Hypercholesterolemic responses in rabbits to selected groups of essential amino acids, **J Nutr,** 1994;124:364-370.
11. Colgan M. **The Sports Nutrition Pocket Guide.** Vancouver: Apple Publications, 1998.
12. Colgan M. **Optimum Sports Nutrition.** Advanced Research Press, New York, 1993.

13. Wang J, Han ZK. Effects of diadzein on muscle growth and some endocrine hormone levels in rats. In Messina MJ, et al(eds). Second International Symposium on the Role of Soy in Preventing and Treating Chronic Diseases. Brussels,Belgium;19 Sept. 1996:45.
14. Coward L, et al. Chemical modification of isoflavones in soy foods during cooking and processing. In Messina MJ, et al(eds). Second International Symposium on the Role of Soy in Preventing and Treating Chronic Diseases. Brussels,Belgium;19 Sept. 1996:70.
15. Slavin JL, et al. Influence of soybean processing, habitual diet and soy dose on urinary isoflavone excretion in humans. In Messina MJ, et al(eds). Second International Symposium on the Role of Soy in Preventing and Treating Chronic Diseases. Brussels, Belgium;19 Sept. 1996:71.

Chapter 47

1. Geller J. **Urology**, 1989,34;Suppl:57-68.
2. Colgan M. **Hormonal Health.** Vancouver, B.C., Apple Publishing, 1996.
3. Tenover JS. **Endocrinol Metab Clin**, 1991;20:893-903.
4. Barlet A, et al. **Wein Klin Wochenschrift,** 1990;102:667-673.
5. Carani C, et al. **Arch Ital Urol,** 1991;63:341-345.
6. Duker EM, et al. **Planta Med**, 1989;55:587.
7. Champault G, et al. **Ann Urol,** 1984;6:407-410.
8. Brackman J. **Curr Ther Res**, 1994;55:776-785.
9. Schneider HJ, et al. **J Forscht Med**, 1995;113:37-40.

Chapter 48

1. Nicholson JP, Case DB. Carboxyhemoglobin levels in New York City runners. **Physician and Sportsmed,** 1983;11:135-138.
2. Stanitski C. Air pollution affects exercise performance. **Clinics in Sports Med**, 1986;4:725-726.
3. Vogel JA, et al. Carbon monoxide and physical work capacity. **Arch Environ Health**, 1972;24:198-203.
4. Murphy P. Coaches lazy about training for smog. **Physician and Sportsmed**, 1984;12:182-183.
5. **Biologic Markers in Immunolgy**, Washington DC: National Research Council, 1992.
6. Raloff J. Air pollution: a respiratory hue and cry. **Science News,** 1991;139:203.
7. Cookson OC, Moffatt MF. Asthma: an epidemic in the absence of infection. **Science,** 1997;275:41-42.
8. Stone R. Immunology: Pollutants a growing threat. **Science,** 1992;256:28.
9. Chow EK, et al. **Environmental Res**, 1981;24:315.

10. Mohammed Z, et al. **FASEB Proc,** 1986;4344.
11. Calabrese E, et al. Influence of dietary vitamin E on susceptibility to ozone exposure. **Bull Environ Contam Toxicol,** 1985;34:417-422.

Chapter 49

1. A, et al. (eds). **Oxyradicals in Molecular Biology and Pathology**. New York, NY: AR Liss, 1988.
2. Harmon D. Aging: A theory based on free radical and radiation chemistry. **J Gerontol**, 1956;11:298-300.
3. Colgan M. **Antioxidants**. Vancouver, BC: Apple Publishing, 1998.
4. Bagchi D, et al. Free radicals and grape seed proanthocyanidin extract: importance in human health and disease prevention. **Toxicology**, 2000;48:187-197.
5. Kitani K, et al (eds). **Pharmacological Intervention In The Aging Process.** New York, NY: New York Academy of Sciences, 1996.
6. Brooks G.A, Fahry TD. **Exercise Physiology**. New York, NY: John Wiley & Sons, 1984.
7. Quintanilha A, In Miguel J, et al. (eds). **Handbook of Free Radicals and Antioxidants**. Boca Raton, FL: CRC Press, 1989.
8. Packer L, et al. (eds). **Biochemical Aspects of Physical Exercise**. Amsterdam: Elsevier, 1985.
9. Pryor WA. **Ann Rev Physiol**, 1986;48:657-667.
10. Gullnick PD, et al. **Eur J Physiol**, 1990;425;407-413.
11. Colgan M. **Optimum Sports Nutrition**. New York, NY: Advanced Research Press, 1993.
12. Karlsson J. Heart and skeletal muscle ubiquinone or CoQ10 as a protective agent against radical formation in man. In Benzi R, Libby B(eds). **Advances in Myochemistry, Eurotext Ltd**, 1987:305-318.
13. Gohill K, et al. Effect of exercise training on tissue vitamin E and ubiquinone content. **J Appl Physiol**, 1987;63:1638-1641.
14. Folkers K, (ed). **Biomedical and Clinical Aspects of Coenzyme Q, Vol Three**. Amsterdam, Elsevier, 1981.
15. Loeschen E, et al. Superoxide radicals as precursors of mitochondrial hydrogen peroxide. **FEBS Letters**, 1974;42:68-72.
16. Maughan RJ, et al. Delayed-onset muscle damage and lipid peroxidation in man after a downhill run. **Muscle and Nerve**, 1989;12:332-336.
17. Tappel A. Will antioxidant nutrients slow the aging process? **Geriatrics**, 1968;23:97-105.
18. Ganther, HE. In Zingaro RA, Cooper WS,(eds). **Selenium**. New York, NY: Van Nostrand, 1974:546-614.
19. Pyke S, et al. Severe depletion of liver glutathione during physical exercise. **Biochem Biophys Res Comm**, 1986;139:926-931.
20. Meister, A. Selective modification of glutathione metabolism. **Science**, 1983;220:474-477.

21. Tsan MF. Modulation of endothelial GSH concentration: effect of exogenous GSH and GSH monoethyl ester. **J Appl Physiol**, 1989;66:1029-1034.

22. Peto R, et al. **Nature**, 1981;290:201-208.

23. Foote, CS, Denny, RW. **J Amer Chem Soc**, 1968,90;6233-6235.

24. Sies H, et al. Antioxidant functions of vitamins. In Sauberlich HE, Machlin LJ (eds). Beyond Deficiency. **Ann NY Acad Sci**, 1992;669:7-20.

25. Di Mascio P, et al. **Methods Enzymol**, 1991;213:429-438.

26. Kennedy, TA, Liebler, DC. **J Biol Chem**, 1992;267:4658-4663.

27. Halliwell B. Free radicals and antioxidants. **Nutr Rev**, 1995;52:253-265.

28. Miguel J, et al. Mitochondrial role in cell aging. **Exp Gerontol**, 1988;15:575-591.

29. Ku HH, et al. Relationship between mitochondrial superoxide and hydrogen peroxide production and longevity of mammalian species. **Free Rad Biol Med**, 1993;15:621-627.

30. Lipoic Acid: The Ideal Antioxidant. **Life Enhancement News.** 1996;11:14-17.

31. Challem J. Is alpha-lipoic acid the ideal antioxidant? **Nutrition Science News**. 1996;8:12-13.

32. Passwater R. **Lipoic-acid: The Metabolic Antioxidant**. New Canaan, CT: Keats Publishing, 1996.

33. Packer L, Witt EH, Tritschler HJ. Alpha-lipoic acid as a biological antioxidant. **Free Radic Biol Med**, 1995;19:227-250.

34. Podda M, Tritschler HJ, Ulrich H, Packer L. Alpha-lipoic acid supplementation prevents symptoms of vitamin E deficiency. **Biochem Biophys Res Commun**. 1994;204:98-104.

35. Han D, Tritschler HJ, Packer L. Alpha-lipoic acid increases intracellular glutathione in human T-lymphocyte Jurkat cell line. **Biochem Biophys Res Commun**, 1995;207:258-264.

36. Constaninescu A, Tritschler H, Packer L. µ-Lipoic acid protects against hemolysis of human erythrocytes induced by peroxyl radicals. **Biochem Mol Biol Int**. 1994;33:669-679.

37. Colgan M. **Protein For Muscle and Strength**. Vancouver, BC: Apple Publishing, 1998.

38. Jacob S, Henriksen EJ, Schiemann Al, et al. Enhancement of glucose disposal in patients with type 2 diabetes by alpha-lipoic acid. **Arzneim Forsch**. 1995;45:872-874.

39. Suziki YJ, Tsuchiya M, Packer L. Lipoate prevents glucose-induced protein modifications. **Free Radic Res Commun**. 1 992;17:211-217.

40. Guillausseau PJ. Pharmacological prevention of diabetic microangiopathy. **Diabete Metabol**. 1994;20:219-228.

41. Ou P, Tritschler HJ, Wolff SP. Thioctic (Lipoic) acid: A therapeutic metal-chelating antioxidant? **Biochem and Pharmacology, Vol. One**, 1995;123:123-126.

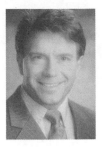

DR. MICHAEL COLGAN, PhD, CCN

Michael Colgan, PhD, CCN, is one of the world's most popular scientific experts in nutrition. He is a best-selling author, and travels the world lecturing on anti-aging, sports nutrition and hormonal health.

From 1971 to 1982, Dr Colgan was a senior member of the Science Faculty of the University of Auckland, where he taught in Human Sciences and conducted research on aging and physical performance. Startling results of his early research convinced him to write his first book for the public, *Your Personal Vitamin Profile (William Morrow, New York)*, during his tenure as a visiting scholar at the Rockefeller University in New York. This revolutionary book rapidly became a definitive guide for accurate, scientifically researched nutritional information.

From 1979 to 1997, Dr Colgan was President of the Colgan Institute of Nutritional Science. He is now Chairman of the Board. The Colgan Institute is a consulting, educational and research facility formed in 1974, primarily concerned with effects of nutrition and exercise on athletic performance, aging and degenerative disease.

With a distinguished reputation for expertise in sports nutrition, Dr Colgan advises hundreds of elite athletes including: track and field Olympians Donovan Bailey, Quincy Watts, Leroy Burrell, Steve Scott, Michelle Burrell, Meredith Rainey Valmon and Regina Jacobs; three-time world boxing champion Bobby Czyz; rowers Francis Reininger and Adrian Cassidy; powerlifting Rick Roberts; two-time world triathalon champion Julie Moss, shooting champion T'ai Erasmus; Australian heavy-weight boxing champion Chris Sharpe; motorcross champion Danny Smith; and bodybuilding champion Lee Labrada, Lee Haney, Laura Creavalle and Lenda Murray.

Professional Memberships

American College of Sports Medicine
New York Academy of Sciences
British Society for Nutritional Medicine
American Academy of Anti-Aging Medicine

Clients

Digital Equipment, Dupont, Twinlabs, Weider Health & Fitness,
US National Institute on Aging,
Price Waterhouse

Other Books by Dr. Colgan

- NEW NUTRITION
- HORMONAL HEALTH
- BEAT ARTHRITIS
- PROTECT YOUR PROSTATE
- NEW POWER PROGRAM
- YOU CAN PREVENT CANCER
- Progress Health Series (6 booklets)
- COLGANChronicles (Newsletter)

Testimonials from Peers

"Listen to this man. He's the best in sports nutrition."
Arthur Lydiard, New Zealand Olympic Coach

"His theoretical development of concepts of preventive nutrition . . . could make an important and unique contribution to the development of preventive medicine in the United States."
Dr Jonas Salk, The Salk Institute

"Crammed with wicked wit and wisdom, irreverent and impertinent, his clear, concise and easily understandable writing is a treat. Ramrod straight, he goes for the jugular of science every time, each conclusion strapped tight to impeccable medical references. And the man himself is a living example of everything he advocates."
Ben Weider, PhD, President, International Federation of Bodybuilders

"The work of the Colgan Institute is an especially valuable contribution of human knowledge."
Dr Andrew Strigner, London

books@applepublishing.com   team@colganinstitute.com   www.colganinstitute.com

INDEX